KONG

Savage Size in 12 Weeks

ALEXANDER BROMLEY

Copyright © 2023 by Alexander Bromley

All rights reserved. This book or any portion thereof may not be reproduced or used in any manner whatsoever without the express written permission of the publisher, except for review and citation purposes.

To my wife Laura, who has spoiled me with her support, love and encouragement, I wouldn't do this without you.

To everybody who has engaged with my content, I couldn't do this without you.

Thank you to Barbell Apparel for being the first company to officially sponsor my channel. I will shamelessly promote their exceptional and unpretentious clothing for as long as they will have me.

Go to www.barbellapparel.com/Bromley for 10% off the best training gear on the market.

Lastly, thank you to YOU!

It is support from readers like you that allow me to create content full-time, and it is IMMENSELY appreciated.

My promise to you is to always offer as much value as possible in anything I publish, sell or promote.

If you enjoyed "KONG: SAVAGE SIZE IN 12 WEEKS", consider checking out my previous full-length books:

<u>BASE STRENGTH: Program Design Blueprint</u>
4.8 Stars on Amazon: 191 Ratings

<u>PEAK STRENGTH: Competitive Performance Roadmap</u>
4.8 Stars on Amazon: 88 Ratings

<u>SUPERIOR DEADLIFT: Technique, Principles, Programming</u>
4.9 Stars on Amazon: 48 Ratings

All are available at www.empirebarbellstore.com or at the Amazon Kindle store here: https://amzn.to/3GcRw2N

These are also available as a courtesy to Patreon members, along with accompanying spreadsheets! https://www.patreon.com/alexanderbromley

TABLE OF CONTENTS

INTRODUCTION 1
LIFTING IS A MESS 3
POPULARITY OF BARBELL SPORTS 11
OVERSPECIALIZATION AND THE NEED FOR VARIETY 15
RON'S STORY: THE PITFALL OF 'AUTHENTIC' TRAINING 23
TIM'S STORY: WHEN DOING WHAT'S ALWAYS
    WORKED STOPS WORKING 31
KONG IS DIFFERENT 39
TENET #1 - WEAK POINTS FIRST 45
TENET #2 - DENSITY 49
TENET #3 - VOLUME 51
TENET #4 - HIGH REPS WITH COMPOUNDS 55
TENET #5 - FATIGUED STRENGTH 61
TENET #6 - LOAD VARIATION 67
TENET #7 - PHASE POTENTIATION 69
PROGRAM BREAKDOWN 71
KONG 77
BLOCK 1 78

BLOCK 2	85
BLOCK 3	93
4 DAY SPLIT	101
BLOCK 1	102
BLOCK 2	103
BLOCK 3	104
HOME GYM 1	105
BLOCK 1	107
BLOCK 2	110
BLOCK 3	112
HOME GYM 2	113
BLOCK 1	115
BLOCK 2	116
BLOCK 3	117

INTRODUCTION

This is the first program that I released that isn't specifically a dedicated strength program. I wrote this to reflect some of the things that I commonly do after the long periods of strength specific training, like in the runs right before World's, but in writing it I also thought about how a lot of this gets neglected by general strength culture in it's pursuit for higher totals at the cost of everything else.

A lot of this e-book is going to be an editorial rant about the state of lifting culture, why it is the way it is, why that's a problem and what you should do about it. A lot of this book is also going to be rote instructional manual on how to run this program as I intended it.

This program first appeared on the BoostCamp app and is still featured as a completely free program on that platform. I had initially thought about dedicating the back half of this book to being a workout journal that would allow you to print out and document all of the sets and reps by hand on paper.

But then I remembered what era I'm living in.

Few people are not using their phones to log their workouts anyways and, given that the BoostCamp app already has KONG loaded up ready to go at no cost to you, it just made sense to direct people there instead.

ALEXANDER BROMLEY

Boostcamp has been a good friend to this channel and I'm really excited for the partnership we have. I look forward to releasing more programs on their application so that I can write more pieces like this. Get KONG on Boostcamp here.

LIFTING IS A MESS

Lifting culture is a mess. The whole fitness industry, including gyms, bodybuilding magazines, supplement companies, the field of exercise science, competitive culture and all of the other organizations that revolve around the pursuit of increasing size, strength and performance……

…are a mess.

Now it has always been a mess. This isn't new or recent. It's been around for as long as people have been able to find ways to get bigger and stronger. So long as there is a continuous influx of new and eager lifters, there is a direct incentive for everyone else involved in lifting culture to have strong opinions about training.

Shit rolls downhill, as they say, so the first-day lifters get lectured by the 6 month veterans who, in turn, watch videos from third year intermediates. They, themselves, pay for coaching from 10 year competitors and all of them stand below the most seasoned coaches and the world champions, many of whom hold the secrets to unchained growth.

And some of whom I wouldn't trust with my nephews little league team.

ALEXANDER BROMLEY

For all of the amazing things about lifting culture, you have to remember that this is very much a consumer-driven field. To those who make money by assisting others in the pursuit of size, strength and performance, the attention of gains-hungry, first-day lifters is their lifeblood. The gym newbies, who at any given time make up the bottom of the fitness-culture iceberg, are the most impressionable and are often eager to get a head start by paying for information, equipment and jugs of powder.

With the advent of social media, the incentive to represent one as an authority no longer just exists for the supplement companies and magazine editors, but also in the average gym goer in a way that it never has before. Today, everyone is an influencer, which means everyone is an authority. And if your'e the new lifter relying on the closest gym hobbyist for sound information, you are no better off than Pinocchio talking to Honest John.

There really is no safe place.

I remember these first influencers, who existed long before 'influencer' was a title. These were the guys who were the most eager to be helpful; they lived in the gym, doing the same exercises with the same weight for decades. I get their rationale: who better to pass the torch than someone who has spent 15 hours per week in a corporate gym weightroom since the Carter administration?

But influence from amateur gym-lifers wasn't all positive…..

Years of chipping away for modest gains, outside of any self-regulating hierarchy of authority, led to an unearned confidence. Many of these well-intentioned gym rats came to believe that their subtle improvements over the years was a sign that they had mastered physical culture. Without any reputable peers checking his work or a stable of trainees working under him to disprove his methods, your average 30 year veteran had no reason to believe that he wasn't qualified to hand out advice.

Personal experience is extraordinarily important.... for you personally. For the rest of population, it is next to worthless. Until you can measure the physical differences between you and everyone else, until you can mark with precision where your limb-length ratios, recovery abilities, pain tolerance and degree of responsiveness land on the bell curve, you have no idea if you grew because of the methods you applied, or in spite of them.

Genetic predisposition is an MFer because the most gifted among us can get really big and really strong without doing much of anything.

If you have the right predisposition, the genes that come by being dealt a better genetic hand can carry you through the most nonsensical, inconsistent training. Forget about training being optimized... some of the best performers barely trained!

I've known great lifters and athletes who have gotten immensely impressive by virtue of doing a lot of work on a semi-regular basis, all with no real effort, planning or direction. I've similarly known top performers that have gotten stupidly big and strong while putting in nothing but effort. No program structure, no tracking of training variables. Just go in, work, and leave.

For this reason, we're left with a paradox when it comes to figuring out what the best modes of training are. Do we follow what the biggest and baddest do? The best performers should have the most keen insight into how to perfect your training. But knowing how much of a role genetics play in physical success, and knowing the fact that the best spots are usually occupied by people with those genes, it seems like trusting the freaks is a sure way to find yourself involved in a method of training that isn't appropriate for the set of genetic tools you have available.

So, do we go the other direction and ignore the outliers, which means ignoring those who did it the best? That leaves us with the lower performers to learn from, which isn't any better. If your rule for finding best training practices involves only looking at what mediocre athletes do, you're going to end up adopting just as many useless rules and bad habits.

I believe that getting over this problem requires building a consensus. While one individual who acheived greatness might have a thing or two to show you about lifting, it's likely enough that that one individual is riding off of some mix of fast genetics and chemical enhancement that their advice might not fit well with you. You have to be skeptical.

But if you add up the training habits of all of the best lifters and coaches and expel the ones that only apply to a select few, you're going to find a list of rules that are universal. The broader principles, the big rocks, followed by the people who have the most amount of experience working with both phenoms and first-timers, don't change much. Once you find them, you will see them present in every program.

Now, finding universal rules is pretty easy. You just turn the dial to 'vague' so that every word of advice is some self-evident bit of common sense. Love your kids. Brush your teeth. Train harder than last time.

The problem is that vague rules lack any teeth. When you reach a certain level of vagueness, you can't apply them to problems in the real world.

Love your kids seems obvious, but it doesn't give you any information on how to navigate the rough terrain of parenting, which involves boundaries and discipline. There has to be counterbalance that corrects course when this initial bit of vagueness goes too far.

Train harder than last time is a common gym truism, and while it's certainly a valid jumping-off point for new lifters to progress their training, it requires more information to be of any use. Taken to its ultimate conclusion, it will run you into over-training, pain, burnout, disillusionment, and it doesn't give you a lick of information about what to do when that happens.

On the other hand, the rules we need to apply can't lose themselves in the details, less they stop becoming relevant to most of the people they are intended for. But they do have to be specific enough that we can actually leverage them to get a better idea of what the hell we're doing.

So I've had 20 plus years as a mediocre lifter, compiling a consensus and trying to carve out these rules so that other mediocre lifters might experience faster progress than myself. I read everything I could, collecting decades worth of bodybuilding magazines and sports journals in the process. I listened to everyone, elite competitor or not, believing that I have more to learn than I do to teach. And over time, as I implemented all of these bits of advice and worldly wisdom into my training, experimenting and program hopping along the way, I started to see how all of these programs fit together, the commonalities they had, and I ended up isolating some principles that seemed to be universal, including principles of when something might work over another.

The thing is, if you're pushing against an external resistance with any amount of effort and you're increasing that resistance over time, you will grow muscle and strength, and probably a bit of endurance. There seems to be more right answers than wrong ones.

That means there are a lot of different modes of training that work. There isn't just one correct path that you have to uncover, you just have to understand the rules you need to follow with whatever path you choose.

Now, breaking training into these universal principles isn't new. Joe Weider did this some 80 odd years ago. Weider's principles are a pretty good starting point. He included principles like range of motion, utilizing sets and implementing progressive overload.

This list got multiple generations of young hopeful bodybuilders off to the right start, but we can improve on those principles a bit.

For strength and performance, you have to be able to predict how you are going to perform on each workout, and that means controlling for stress and recovery. That's a problem with strength training that we often run into with our programming, that doing whatever, while it might work in the short term, it runs you into a wall because you can't anticipate when the work you did to grow you in the first place suddenly becomes too much to bounce back from.

For KONG, I'm going to talk about the things that lead to unrestricted, overgrown levels of muscular development. These are the big things that, implemented by themselves are usually enough to transform the physiques of young lifters but, when we pair them together, the whole becomes greater than the sum of its parts.

Once you get a handle on how to reliably experience this type of growth, increasing strength is just a matter of when, not if.

We're going to talk bout movement selection. Everybody knows this to be important, but no matter how self-evident it seems, it always bears repeating.

We're going to talk about the role of compound movements in building size and strength,

We're going to talk about the role of high reps, high volume, high density, and high fatigue in creating a massive stimulus for growth.

We're going to talk about phase potentiation and how to plan your training so that the qualities you develop today directly improves your training next week.

We're going to talk about variety and novelty and how important they are in keeping you engaged, growing and free from burnout.

So grab some steel wool, latex gloves and a bucket of bleach and let's start cleaning this mess up.

POPULARITY OF BARBELL SPORTS

I think it's great that power lifting and barbell strength sports have grown immensely in popularity in the last 10 to 15 years. And I'm not just saying that as somebody who makes my money telling people how and when to lift. There are numerous benefits that strength training has to offer the general population, aside from individuals looking better, feeling better and establishing that they have an agency in changing their life at the deepest level.

It's a generally noble mission for any society to have a strong, capable population who knows their way around their own body, just as you would want your motorists to have passed basic Driver's Ed.

A nation of lifters will be more resilient and more capable. They will have stronger bones and their elderly populations will be much less likely to succumb to breaks caused by osteoporosis. Something as simple as reinforcing someone's ability to get out of a chair into their eighties ensures that they're not going to become bed bedridden as early, and that buys them years, if not decades.

A nation of lifters will live longer and experience more vitality for the years that they are alive.

Now, the growth in strength sports, especially powerlifting, can be credited to two things. First is CrossFit introducing millions of people to the barbell. Second is the changes in the basic rules of power lifting that ditched the sweaty, bloated, pre-diabetic, squat-suit wearing stereotype that turned the sport into an inaccessible freak show through the 80s, 90s and 2000s.

Now, don't get me wrong, as a strongman competitor, I have very fond memories of when my sport was an inaccessible freak show. We would gather next to the storage unit that we used to hoard all of our makeshift equipment and inconvenience just about everyone by rolling out giant tires, 100' long manilla ropes and countless dozens of 45lb plates into the street as we claimed it as our runway. We loved that we were giving a collective middle finger to everyone who wasn't us; something as simple as being a motorist headed to work was enough to separate you from I. We were so used to being separate that we revelled in the looks of 'WTF' that we would get as we dragged giant chains and ran with kegs on our shoulders. We were each "off" in our own way, awkward, outcast and willing to use personal suffering under the strain of a yoke or sandbag as a coping mechanism.

For the die hards and first adopters of the sport, nothing beat it.

But as it turns out, if you want other people to join your club you have to turn the music down and put on some pants.

The barbell lifts that make up powerlifting (the squat, bench, and deadlift) are not only amazing developmental tools with a relatively short learning curve, but they're the most accessible tools for building strength you can find. If you want a crash course in the barbell, you need only seek out any one of the countless corporate gyms that exist all over the world that will give you access for $10 a month.

The natural, raw movement in powerlifting has redifined the image of strength sports and now features more lifters who have physiques that are somewhat desirable to the mainstream. And because success in the sport no longer requires learning how to use triple-ply, Kevlar lifting suits and finding a team of people that can actually help you in and out of them, more and more people are able to participate in powerlifting simply by going to their local corporate gym and spending some time in the squat rack.

CrossFit got this whole thing started by getting everybody excited about the barbell. They were smart enough to feature basic barbell lifts as a staple in their boot camp style conditioning classes, because the barbell is an effective developmental tool, sure, but also because it represented a bit of counterculture at the time. There was something new and interesting about barbell training, especially the Olympic lifts, which were held in higher esteem as a more posh and formal form of lifting but less known by the general public. This immediately gave everybody involved a mild sense of superiority, which is the best way to grow an army of loyal enthusiasts.

A big chunk of CrossFitters started doing the odd Olympic lifting or powerlifting meets in compliance of the Crossfit mantra of being ready for anything. Many eventually fell in love with these sports and realized that lifting weights normally was just as, if not more, fun than killing yourself in a 20 minute barn-burning, metabolic conditioning workout.

Then strongman began to grow, which further helped bridge the gap between 'functional fitness' and pure strength training. The appeal of these sports led to previously unseen levels of mass participation and popularity.

Now, this is all great for all of the people that have been chanting for years, "We need to grow the sport!" Boy, did we and how.

But that leaves us with a problem; in getting sold to the masses it is inevitable for the culture, which was so unique in it's abililty to create wide-sweeping transformation in it's members, to get watered down. Eventually, important features that made the thing valuable to begin with get cast aside in the name of just getting more signups.

For those who plan on training long term and have lofty performance goals, I mean those who can see themselves training for 20 years or more and believe they ought to be able to make steady improvements for the duration of that time, some attention should be paid to making sure that their training fits that goal. That's done by making sure it A.) has direction and B.) is sustainable. This is where all new lifters fall into their first trap, their first plateau, where by virtue of working hard and growing without any concern for A or B, they think they have 'figured it out' and are lulled into a false security about their knowledge of what it takes to get bigger and stronger continuously.

It's somewhere around the late novice/early intermediate stage that this happens. This is the stage where you can see yourself being competitive, like a mirage on the desert, but aren't quite there yet and aren't sure when you will be. At this stage, you start to experience your first speed bumps, where several sessions don't lead to immediate increases in strength, and then eventually you find yourself in a rut where nothing budges for months or, God help you, years.

OVERSPECIALIZATION AND THE NEED FOR VARIETY

It's important to talk about overspecialization because the program I'm giving you is written specifically with the average, 'overspecialized' lifter in mind. If it works for you, it's likely because you've spent so much time doing the exact opposite of this that you were simply just due for a change.

The big problem with CrossFit and powerlifting getting people involved in barbell sports is that the barbell was eventually placed on a pedestal. It became the altar you prayed at every time you went to church. It was romanticized, deified, and because of that, the disciples became hesitant to spend any time or attention giving their effort to another, lesser mode of training.

The thing you have to understand is that barbell movements are extremely effective, but they're also extremely limited. I will always maintain barbell workouts in my workout, but as I've gotten more advanced over the years I had to get very aggressive with how I incorporated secondary exercises to fix weaknesses and make sure that I could continue to grow.

You might find that barbell squatting blows up your legs and increases your strength after just a few months but over many years you might find that your quads just don't respond the way that your other friend's do. Or you might find that your shoulders don't grow quite as well from benching.

The solution to this isn't more stubborn specificity and a narrow focus on the same 3 things. Rather, it is a multi-varied approach that doesn't leave any stone unturned. In short, the solution is variety.

Variety is essential for long-term continued growth. It makes you well-rounded, sure, but it also ensures that the thing that you're doing isn't going to become so routine and monotonous that your body forgets it's supposed to grow as a result of experiencing it.

Variety can mean a lot of different things, so it's important we put some boundaries around it.

Firstly, it is not simply jumping around from workout to workout, letting the last thing you read from your favorite underground fitness blog determine what is done on any given day. 'Variety' isn't approval to do whatever the hell pops into your head or to ditch your commitments every time your eye catches a shiny new e-book. You need to work things long enough to get good at them.

I think… no, I KNOW…. that periods of specialization are incredibly valuable but every unit of time you spend past the point of greatest returns is going to yield diminished returns. So, if you like doing the same three barbell lifts and the same basic rep range and the same basic split year in, year out, you can pat yourself on the back that you're being very strength specific. You can even be sure you are going to get very strong in the beginning. But those strength gains are inevitably going to slow down and then eventually they're going to stop altogether. Time, effort, and wear is going to accumulate on your body and you won't have a lot to show for it. Worst of all, you're going to come to absolutely hate your training.

The variety that I'm talking about involves letting yourself go through different periods of training where you prioritize different things beyond that next all-time PR. The best representation of all of this is going to come in phase potentiation, where you are deliberately spending weeks if not months in pursuit of one particular goal, only to take a step back, reevaluate and apply the progress made there to making better something else.

For most of you, you don't have to walk a razor thin line with phase potentiation. Just pick a method of training you like and commit yourself to it long enough to get good at it. Then and only then, try something else that uses a different approach to get to your goals. As long as effort is present along with the desire to improve (and as long as these program decisions aren't coming out of left field) you should be able to stack together successful blocks of training and experience continued growth for a long period of time.

More importantly, you should be able to learn which exercises, ranges, and modes of training you tend to respond to the best. You want to have not one, but multiple, go-to programs that you know are reliable so that you can bounce back and forth to one when the other becomes stagnant.

Variety should entail a mix of exercises, compounds and isolations, free weights and machines and should involve the full spectrum of different energy systems. Regardless of what you want to be true, you are not better off for not doing any cardiovascular work. Strength is only as useful as your ability to express it, and it turns out you can't express it very well if you turn purple and flop on your back after 15 seconds of effort.

You want to do a variety of rep ranges. You want to incorporate a variety of tempos and positions. You want to temper yourself to different demands so that you have fewer weaknesses and so that you are more adaptable.

If you do eventually decide to dedicate all of your effort to becoming the next great powerlifter, your dedication will be set up for success in a way that makes your eventual dominance a certainty.

Variety is so important in creating greater potential for success that it is the cornerstone principle in the training of young athletes in virtually every sport that exists. It's been known for the better part of a century that young lifters and athletes should be exposed to variety that tests and develops them in different ways. Off of that foundation that you can have them specialize later in their career, but the peak that they can potentially reach is only going to be as high as the width of their base.

If youth athletes who aren't yet experienced enough to justify highly specialized training, should go through varied movements with body weight exercises, dumbbells, unilateral work and the like, then certainly young lifters would benefit the same.

So, variety is important. It's important when you start and it's important in some capacity through the rest of your training career. Remember, you are not better for being a one trick pony.

When I put Kong together, I had one thing in mind: I wanted people to be able to take a quantum leap forward to replace the inches of progress that they were scraping out with ball breaking workouts. I wanted to outline the catalyst for a monumental shift forward that was going to propel them miles ahead of where they were. To do that with so many people, there has to be some universal problem, something that is easy to identify, easy to fix and that applies to most in the audience.

Plenty of those problems exists in general lifting culture and Kong addresses them.

I've written extensively about overspecialization and how focusing on your few favorite pet barbell lifts can lead to stagnation and the creation of weak areas, in addition to causing eventual burnout. That represents a big problem among modern lifters and simply taking a step back to revisit some older, broader methods of training can be hugely productive, not just at giving yourself a break, but in shoring up the deficits that are holding you back.

Kong is anti-specialization. It acknowledges the connection between size and strength and the truth that, for the average person, the most accessible way to increase strength is to add muscle to their frame. It builds off the belief that any one individual is going to be the absolute strongest when they can hold the most amount of muscle.

Now, forget about turning into an absolute mass monster. Surely, some of you might want to go that route and this is certainly a step in that direction. But I know many of you don't.

Anybody who has a thought of some grotesque bodybuilder and thinks, "Ew, I'd never want to be that muscular", don't worry. You're not in danger of going through the first block and waking up at a bulbous 300 pounds and in need of a new wardrobe.

If at any point you look in the mirror or the scale and don't like what you see, you can cut bait. Even when muscle growth happens radically, it happens pretty slowly. With something as difficult as tricking your body into synthesizing grams of protein into kilograms of new tissue it doesn't really need, you can't afford to take a "well, a little but not too much" approach. That tends to work out about as good as doing nothing at all.

For those of you who just want to find your ideal body type, whether it's the 50lbs needed to fill out your frame or the 5lbs needed to be a little stronger and more conditioned, this will get you there faster.

Kong relies on modes of training that were historically used by some of the most advanced lifters around, modes which have been largely abandoned in today's training culture. Now, many people do this while hiding behind the shield of specificity.

"I want to be strong, and that's not strength specific, therefore it's beneath me."

If you commit long enough to be able to see the benefits that this type of training can have (regardless of your goals), it becomes so obvious how beneficial it is that you wonder why you never did it to begin with.

Now, if this training is so effective, why do so few people do it? That's a really good question and I think the obvious answer is that it is somewhat of a bastardized training approach. It doesn't fit cleanly with one category, with one sport, with one identity.

I'm convinced that most people avoid the small work because it's an affront to their manufactured identity of 'strength athlete' or 'barbell specialist', which illustrates how many will put a superficial association with 'strong things' ahead of actually becoming strong. I'm sure it also gets avoided because it's uncomfortable and requires understanding of how to handle a completely different type of strain. I have worked with professional strongman competitors who would kill themselves completing a max deadlift but wouldn't get within 10 reps of failure on a leg press.

People are eager when they're new to glob onto the culture that they're immersing themselves in. They use it to add to their personal identity and establish clout. Pledging allegiance to one brand establishes connectedness to something bigger than themselves and satisfies a need for validation.

Strength training appeals to insecure individuals in need of some substantive transformation, a situation I identify with on a very personal level. For that reason, it tends to transcend the label of 'hobby' and become very, very connected to the lifter's sense of self (not with all of us, I'm sure, but enough of us as to merit a paragraph or two on it). As long as training is part of self-help, that will always be true. That's not a dig and it's not all bad; there are worse ways to find stability, confidence and leverage in the world. But it needs to be ackowledged to avoid the bad conclusions that ideology and personal identity can lead to.

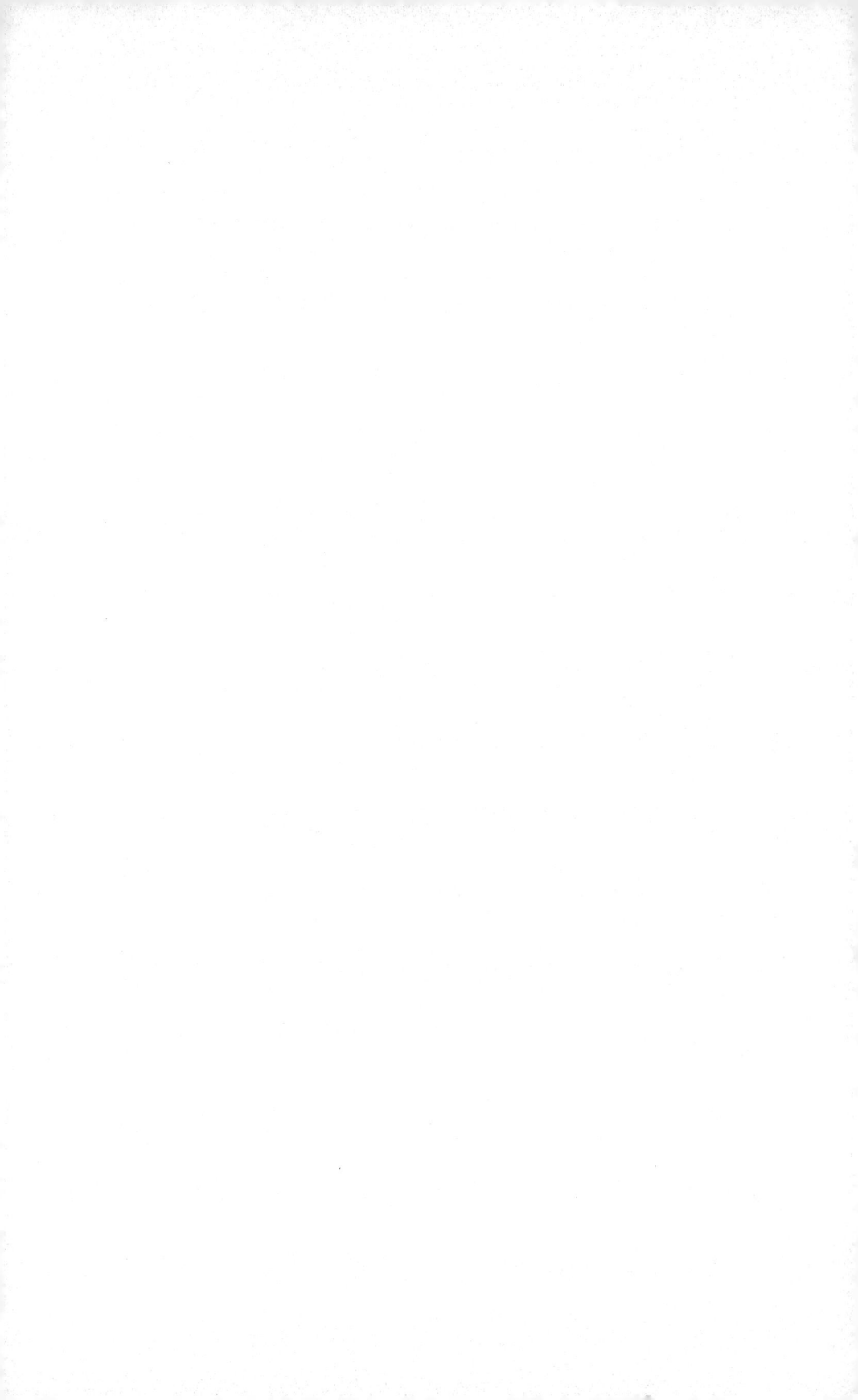

RON'S STORY: THE PITFALL OF 'AUTHENTIC' TRAINING

Ron was a member of Empire Barbell, the gym that I owned in Redlands, California from 2016 to 2022.

He had found us because he was eager to get into what felt like a more authentic powerlifting gym. He was an athletic guy, about six foot with the build of a solid 220lb powerlifter or middleweight strongman. He was athletic looking, but was actually stronger than his build might suggest. He had a lot of potential.

Now, in getting hooked on strength acquisition as a hobby, Ron ended up becoming fixated on the teachings of Louie Simmons and Westside Barbell. He would routinely engage me in arguments, though they wouldn't ever really get past the point of simple regurgitations of the last Louie-ism he had read.

Walk with the lame, develop a limp.

Cheetahs don't have to warm up before they hunt.

Big isn't strong. Strong is strong.

...and the like.

It often felt like the same type of blind reciting of source material that fanatics use when they're trying to use their religious text to tell you why their religious text is correct.

I would insist that the success experienced by those that ran the system wasn't due to the things that he thought they were (like the magic of ME/DE splits, accomodating resistance or the rejection of basic periodization) and that, as a method of training, it wasn't appropriate for somebody in his situation.

Conjugate style training is best done in a team setting or, at the very least, under the eye of somebody that's had a lot of success running it. There's a big learning curve when you're swapping movements every week because every movement isn't created equal. There's an art-form to picking movements that will carry over to the main lifts and you won't acquire that skill until you've been around the block a few times.

There's also an inclination a lot of lifters have to spend all of their time on the max effort and dynamic effort work and sandbag the repetition stuff and the accessory work. And hardly anybody takes the GPP.

But I digress. I watched Ron cycle through his pet movement variations every week. He was focused on building his deadlift up and he seemed to avoid squat work. He would say it was because he cared more about his deadlift, but I know it was because the squat was an awkward movement for his leggy frame.

So he would go from banded deadlifts to rack pulls to good mornings to every other variation he could think of. In fact, I don't think I ever saw him do the same variation twice. He took a similar approach for his bench press, although he had to keep one foot on the brake because of shoulder issues that sidelined him.

I couldn't be too judgmental because it made sense to me. He was a new lifter who became attached to the most recognizable brand in the game. Even though Westside/Conjugate training is not done by the overwhelming majority of successful powerlifters, it still commands a huge following and a reputation for being an innovative force in lifting culture as a whole.

Westside used a particular style to brand itself, primarily the black and white image of a jacked, bald powerlifter, spitting, and screaming as they strained under a barbell loaded with impossible amounts of weights in a messy underground gym. It had a sheen of authenticity that was appealing to new initiates. I understood why Ron got taken in by it.

12 months to the day from Ron joining the gym, he decided to do a test to see what fruits a year of his own loyal Westside conjugate adaptation had yielded.

His bench didn't improve at all, which wasn't surprising given the shoulder issues he had with benching. He was very optimistic, but because he hadn't done the main lifts in 12 months or more, he had no barometer of what to expect.

His bench didn't improve at all and I'll never forget the look of defeat and disillusionment on his face. I had to work to choke back the words "I EFFING told you."

His shoulders were buggy and he did kind of a half compromise where he would follow the rotation of exercises but keep effort down according to how he felt that day. It was the worst combination of managing pain and pushing past it and he didn't getting much out of the pressing days as a result.

His squatting was an accessory to his deadifting and, because his long legs made it an awkward movement, I felt that he wasn't doing enough to develop skill and comfort in weakest, most awkward position.

As far as the deadlift... well, of all the things I've seen lead to really, really big pulls, max effort singles on a weekly basis with a huge rotating stable of movements just isn't one of them. I'm not saying it couldn't have worked out that way, but I'm am saying the art of movement selection required experience that he didn't have.

So at the end of the day... nothing on his bench, nothing on his squat, 20 pounds on his deadlift. He was dejected. After a year of spinning his wheels, applying all of his effort towards what he thought was the most authentic version of strength training, the most specialized, legit, hardcore program he could find, he realized that it didn't do a damn thing for his numbers.

I finally convinced him to follow a program of mine, which is listed below. The approach is simple: the same lifts, twice a week with an emphasis on building skill and confidence and adapting to a lot of work.

With him, I strongly felt that he needed more time on the same lifts and that just existing in those awkward positions for more time every week would build confidence and he would actually be able to apply himself to bigger squats. He needed practice reps and a lot of them and was looking for any reason to avoid them. Instead, he lived for the gratification that came from the one-and-done max effort sets. He would spend way too much time fidgeting over band tension charts and wave progressions for the speed work. I had reason to believe that, with just a dash of movement specificity, he would hit a PR just from the psychological benefit of being familiar with the movement.

I gave him a five week cycle and stretched it out to 10 by having him run it twice. It was very simple: a heavy day where he worked up to a top set of reps, not singles, and then an alternate day that involved repeating sets of high reps.

The same movement was repeated every week, accessory work was made a priority and fatigue was built up from high reps. No bands. No accommodating resistance. No rotation of movements.

Just do this thing long enough to get good at it, and then repeat. Ron's improvements were nothing short of incredible

To deal with his shoulder. I had him stop trying to find a magic bench variation that would skyrocket his bench without causing pain and instead programmed nothing but overhead.

ALEXANDER BROMLEY

	Week 1	Week 2	Week 3
Day 1			
Bench Press	3x6 @ 70% last set max reps	5x6 @75% last set max reps	4x4 @ 78% last set max reps
Wide Grip Bench Press	3x10	5x8-10	8x8
Inverted Row (use body weight) superset w/	3x10	4x10	5x12
DB Fly	3x15	4x15	5x12
One Arm DB Row superset w/ DB Pullover	3x15	4x15	5x12
Skull Crushers superset w/ Barbell Curl	3x15	4x15	5x15
Concentration Curl superset w/ Tricep Kickback	3x15	4x15	5x15
Day 2			
Squat	3x5 @ 70% last set max reps	6x5 @75% last set max reps	4x4 @ 78% last set max reps
Front Squat	3x10	5x8-10	8x8
Romanian DL (5 sec negative)	3x6	4x6	6x5
Single-Leg Press superset with	3x15	4x15	5x12
single-leg Hamstring Curl	3x15	4x15	5x12

	Week 4	Week 5	Week 6 DELOAD	
	3x3 @ 83% last set max reps	1x3+ @ 88 last set max reps	3x3 @ 75%	
	4x6	3x5	3x5 @ RPE 6	
	4x15	3x15	2x12	
	4x12	3x10	2x8	
	4x12	3x10	2x8	
	4x12	3x12	2x10	
	4x12	3x12	2x10	
	3x3 @ 83% last set max reps	1x3+ @ 88 last set max reps	3x3 @ 75% last set max reps	
	4x6	3x5	3x5 @ RPE 6	
	5x4	3x4	2x4 @ RPE 6	
	4x12	3x10	2x8	
	4x12	3x10	2x8	

	Week 1	Week 2	Week 3
Day 3			
Close Grip Bench (forefinger on ring)	Max 5 err on no missed reps	Max 3	Max 5
Incline Bench Press	3x6	4x6	8x5
Dips superset with	3 x max reps	4 x max reps	5 x max reps
CG Pulldown	3x8-10	4x8-10	5x8-10
Wide Bent Row superset w/ DB Lateral Raise	3x10-12	4x10-12	5x10
French Press superset w/ Alternating DB Curl	3x10-12	4x10	5x10
Bench Dips superset w/	3 x max reps	4 x max reps	5 x max reps
Hammer Curl	3x10-12	4x10-12	5x10
Day 4			
Pause Squat	Max 5 keep technical ceiling	Max 3	Max 5
Deficit Deadlift (2", stand on mats or plates)	3x6 @ 85%	4x6 @ 70%	5x5 @ 75%
Alternating DB Lunge	3x12/12	4x10/10	5x10/10
Back Extension w/ pause at top	3x12 body weight	4x12 body weight	5x10 add weight

	Week 4	Week 5	Week 6
	Max 2	Max 1	Top single @ RPE 6-7
	4x4	3x3	3x3 @ RPE 6
	4 x max reps	3 x max reps	2 x 12
	4x8	3x6	2x6
	4x8	3x8	2x8
	4x8-10	3x8	2x8
	4 x max reps	3 x max reps	2 x max reps
	4x8	3x8	2x8
	Max 2	Max 1	Top single @ RPE 6-7
	4x4 @ 80%	85% x max reps	2x3 @ 75%
	4x8/8	3x8/8	2x8/8
	4x10 add weight	3x8 add weight	2x8 add weight

He went from being able to incline bench 225 for sets of 8 to 10 with pain to being able to push press 225 for just as many, pain free. His squat jumped over a hundred pounds, having failed at a 405 attempt after his year of conjugate and ultimately hitting 465 for reps at the end this new program.

As for his deadlift, I don't think I had ever seen him go over 3 reps before this. While that fed into his strength as an explosive puller in the beginning, that limited approach to building his deadlift got stale really fast. After a few weeks of actually doing some work, his labored 405 for 10 was replaced with a no-bones-about-it 455 for 12. His deadlifting ability had turned into a different animal altogether.

There are multiple examples of this type of training revelation that I've witnessed over the years, where the lifter reluctantly commits to the one thing they need (which is always the one thing they hate doing) and gets floored by the results. But this one stood out. It's rare that I get such a satisfying conclusion to what starts as an emphatic ideological argument.

Ron still wasn't sold completely and he would still be the Louie apologist whenever the topic came up. I think some of that was pride and not wanting to backtrack on the hill that he spent so much time bleeding out on (which all but it reaffirmed what I already knew about training culture and identity).

The secret to growth, and I mean quick, nasty growth, is a lot of effort over a lot of sets with compound movement for a lot of reps. If you apply yourself to that, you will transform, you will turn into something else. That's the only hill you should be dying on.

TIM'S STORY: WHEN DOING WHAT'S ALWAYS WORKED STOPS WORKING

See, bodybuilders have a very distinct style and it doesn't really matter which bodybuilding camp you fall into. To build the competitive package, the entire body has to be hit evenly and that's only done with a lot of smaller movements. So anybody who calls themself a bodybuilder is going to be doing a whole host of different free-weight, machine and cable exercises.

The barbell takes a hard back seat in bodybuilding training, if it isn't removed altogether. Physical symmetry takes precedent over everything else, so even if you can argue that you're sacrificing the benefit of load by putting barbell lifts later in the workout, the well rounded development you get by putting the smaller movements first can potentially outweigh that. This is true even for a dedicated strength athlete.

Scores of people who do their heavy barbell stuff first still suffer deficiencies in vital accessory muscle groups that hold them back from their true potential. Bodybuilders as a group simply don't have that problem.

As valuable as this feature of physique-focused training is, it can be taken too far. Read on.

Tim joined my gym in 2016 and we became fast friends.

I enjoyed shooting the shit with him as much as anybody about the ins and outs of training because few people had as much passion for training and understand really what goes into long term lifting success.

Tim had identified a bodybuilder his entire life. He became enamored with that aspect of physical culture at a very young age, deciding before he was even a teenager that he was going to do anything it took to be competitive on that stage. He started paying attention to the greats, tracking down the most muscular guys in the gym and figuring out how they structured their training, what they focused on in each working set and what their diets consisted of. Tim ended up falling into a decades long pattern of grueling, isolation based body building workouts and eating like a monk. Everybody knew when Tim had arrived because the gym would fill with the smell of the tilapia that he just microwaved and the screams he would let loose while punishing himself on the leg extension machine.

The principles that Tim abided by in his training prioritized effort, but in a specific way where you aim to keep tension on the muscle so that you feel it every rep. Early on, he was taught to focus on the squeeze of the contraction, to lower the weight under control, to stay in a specific range of motion, usually short of lockout and short of a full stretch that traps blood and doesn't allow metabolites to be flushed. By doing this, the idea is that you can keep mechanical tension on the muscle, reach a deeper level of fatigue and create a better growth stress.

For instance, if you do a set of squats without any attention to which muscles are working, which muscles derive the primary growth benefit is going to primarily come down to how you're built. But if you know how to position your toes, where to shift your weight, how far forward to push your knees, how to pulse in the mid-range of the rep, you can ensure that your target muscle (let's say, your quads) has to work harder than anything else. And when today isn't just squat day but *quad* day, those variations are extremely important.

Now, Tim had an impressive physique. He had round muscle bellies, low body fat and it was evident to anybody from the moment he walked in the room that he had spent many years of his life hammering away in the gym.

The problem came when Tim entered into a national qualifier. He had spent 12 weeks dieting down, getting absolutely peeled as he put in all of his years of dedicated, obsessive work towards the pursuit of bodybuilding glory into one all-out prep.

He showed up against the one other contender in his class, a guy who looked like he had been doing this for some time and was ready to do it at a higher level. Both Tim and his competitor were large. They were full. They had impressive definition, and it was evident that they didn't leave anything on the table during their prep.

Of all of the classes, Tim and his competitor had the longest showdown. The judges were obviously torn, having them cycle through the same poses again and again, having them stand side by side and mulling over their performances much longer than any of the other competitors

From from the back, Tim had him absolutely whipped. Not surprising given that the man lived and died by chins, rows and more chins. He included in his back training everything under the sun, from heavy cheated T-bar rows through limited ranges of motion to isolated cable work, to pulse reps and drop sets, and of course, the movement he would never exclude from a workout, pull-ups.

Tim had one of the biggest and most separated backs of anybody on stage that night.

But when it came to the front poses, where you could see how the size and definition of the upper body balanced with the proportions of the lower body, Tim fell short and that inevitably cost him the show. Tim's legs were muscular, sure, but they were long and thin, almost aerodynamic. They didn't have the girth that one expects from the legs of the best bodybuilders in the sport. They didn't even match the impressive development of his own upper body.

Now, I had watched Tim train for years at that point and I'd seen how he handled his workouts with his most impressive body parts: his upper back, his pecs, his arms.

He would routinely make increases in weight, trying to hang with the other guys in the gym, and got strong in the process. It wasn't uncommon to see Tim benching 315 for reps and I even saw him get over 400 pounds a couple of times. Not bad for a guy that was 175 on stage.

On leg day, however, he would hyper fixate on the 'feeling' of his quadriceps. Now, part of me believes it's because Tim, along with most bodybuilders, are masochists at heart and they condition themselves to work through their personal/emotional baggage with twisted stuff like leg press drop-sets and 100 rep lunges.

There's a cleansing, almost spiritual effect to this type of work. To many, only when the acid produced around the muscles during forced reps of leg extensions makes you consider going home and never doing this again, can you really say you've trained.

You learn to rate the effectiveness of your training on the pain experienced during. When you're using advanced techniques common to bodybuilders (like negatives, drop sets, forced reps, partials, rest-pause, supersets and the like) and especially when you apply that with positioning changes that are designed to put the stress right in the belly of the muscle, well, the pain is incredible and it's the thing that limits most people from their full potential.

At the end of the day, the guy who's going to be the biggest, the densest and the most shredded is going to be the guy who is willing to suffer more than the other guy. You have to be a little off to do this, and Tim and I would both say that Tim is a little off.

As valuable as pain tolerance is and as many lessons as it can teach you, pain for the sake of it isn't the point. In all of his world-ending leg workouts, Tim would refuse to add weight. He would exclaim that when he squatted more, he wouldn't feel it in his legs so he thought it was worthless.

Now, this made a certain type of sense. I've been squatting for weight my whole life and I couldn't tell you which muscles I felt on the biggest squat sets I've ever done. It becomes more about the movement pattern and which muscles take the beating is going to depend on individual factors, like how long your legs are, how far back your hips go, what your knees and ankles are doing and so on.

So Tim, having long legs and being somewhat of an awkward squatter, would hyper fixate on what he was or wasn't feeling during each squat set. For that reason, he never liked going over 225.

Now, it wasn't for fear of the weight and it certainly wasn't because going heavy was somehow harder than what he was already doing. The efforts he put out with 20 to 30% of his training max was as nauseating to watch as it was impressive and anybody in the room would be hard pressed to make the case that his methods were somehow the easy way out.

Even with his clients, he was infamous for having them start with a hundred reps of body weight lunges then go into their squatting workout, followed by squatting variations, unilateral work, leg presses for endless reps and forced sets. And then when you thought you didn't have anything left in the tank... right back into squats.

No, it wasn't work ethic or pain tolerance. He was obsessed with the idea that the secret to growth came from having a deep connection to the muscle, so he emphasizing the sensation of stress rather than the mathematics of progressive overload.

From where I'm standing, a man with an impressive upper body who is used to handling a certain amount of weight is not going to have a lower body to match if the weight he uses in a typical set of squats doesn't get within 100lbs of what he handles in a typical bench workout. I've seen Tim bench 365lbs more than I've seen him get 275lbs on the squat bar, so it's no wonder when he stepped on stage that his legs were the weak point.

This was confirmed when he talked to a mentor and close confidant, a female pro bodybuilder and world record holder powerlifter who trained at a local gym he frequented. When picking her brain about how to prep for his upcoming meet, she gave him the same pill that I was carefully trying to get him to swallow: unless weight increases became a priority, he was never going to see the growth that he wanted.

Long before all this, there was about a six month period where I got Tim on the strongman wagon and he ran through a couple of my strength programs. I've seen him bang out 500 pound squats for sets of five: no wraps, no belt, ass touching the floor and with reps to spare. It should go without saying that Tim was looking beefy around that time but in typical bodybuilder fashion, he looked past the growth and just saw the cracks in his physique. Paranoia grew the longer he was away from the mode of training he had done for 20 years, until he abandoned the heavy weight, cut his calories and went right back to blood boiling endurance fests with light weights.

Now, Tim has good genetics by anybody's standard but he's not a freak. The freaks, the outliers, the ones on an immense amount of PEDs who grow just from looking at a weight, might be able to get away with such a routine as long as they're well fed and not skipping any injections.

But unless you're that one in 10,000, you don't have the luxury of leaving anyting on the table. There's no doubt in my mind that something as simple as a few sets of threes and fives, progressed consistently over time and followed by all of the other insanity that he was used to, would have made Tim's legs the show-stealers rather than his Achilles' heel.

This reaffirms something that I always knew and that's that the biggest and the baddest are going to be the ones that commit to not leaving any stone unturned. Having a pet method of training is important because you need to be able to like what you do, especially if you are going to invest your life in it. But success, paradoxically, only comes to those who are willing to prioritize all the things they don't like. If you just lean on your simple preferences, then you have to accept that how developed you get and how well rounded you are is going to be little more than a crapshoot.

KONG IS DIFFERENT

Follow any bodybuilder around for a workout, whether he's a golden-era disciple of volume or a new age, high intensity, Mike Mentzer fanatic. You're still going to see similar exercises worked to a very, very high point of fatigue with a lot of reps, total work and total effort being applied.

As you move across the spectrum, away from size and into the realm of strength and performance, this flips on its head. Strength focused sports like powerlifting and Olympic weightlifting rely on lower rep ranges to maximize the development of strength-specific qualities. In fact many will stick with low reps exclusively, replacing sets of 12, 10, 8 reps with nothing but triples or lower.

The benefit is that you get to treat the barbell movements like a skill, in addition to creating neurological adaptations that allow for more force production. More efficiency means more weight on the bar in training and on the platform, more weight means more strength adaptations, and the cycle continues.

Since skill development is such an important factor with powerlifters and strength-fanatics, it makes sense that some modes of training dedicate most of the workout to practice-reps with those lifts. The obsession with specificity causes the performance-focused lifter to avoid anything that doesn't draw a straight line to their one rep max, so smaller accessory work and high rep sets get left by the wayside.

The approach used in Kong blends elements of these brands of training in a way that doesn't fit one particular identity. Its closest relative on the spectrum would be 'powerbuilding', a type of training that respects the necessity of being skilled in developing strength in the barbell movements while also paying attention to the type of broad developmental work that is a trademark of the most muscular people on the planet.

The idea of powerbuilding is, and I think this is about as self-evident as it gets, that these two things together only reinforce each other, and that you get the greatest possible return in terms of size developed and strength potentially expressed by effectively combining these priorities. There have been a lot of greats who have trained like this before; it certainly isn't a new approach.

There's a blog called 70's Big that was run by Green Beret Justin Lascek that paid homage to this type of lifter. The inspiration for the site was the type of physique and presence strength athletes had in the 70's, which isn't quite as common today (which is strange considering how many more people train specifically for powerlifting today than back then).

The argument can be made that there were fewer walls put up between different strength sports back then. Bodybuilders would dabble in Olympic lifting, using rough variations of cleans, high pulls and push presses in addition to their preacher curls and sissy squats.

Barbell clubs usually featured members who were so enamored with lifting for the sake of lifting that they wanted to know everything about all of the different nooks and crannies that make up physical culture. And at the time, the pool of participants was so small that there really wasn't enough room to separate you from the other iron heads based on petty differences in training tastes. The fact of being in a gym and lifting with a competitive spark was enough to connect you to whichever other type of athlete you happened to be around.

World's Strongest Man, starting in 1977, epitomized the free-flow spirit of this era: it was made specifically to contest how bodybuilders, powerlifters, football players and the like would fare out of their comfort zone given odd, unfamiliar tasks. Now, it's such a specialized endeavor that fans throw a fit when a world record holder in another barbell sport, a legitimate claimant to the title of 'World's Strongest Man', gets an invite to a big show without winning an amateur backyard show first.

Simply put, it was a less divisive time, so it's not surprise that when you look back you see a mishmash of training principles making up the routines of the strongest and most muscular people on the planet.

Anybody can look up the programs carried out by the likes of Bill Kazmaier, Doug Young and Roger Estep. Hard work with heavy weights followed by lots of effort with lots of different supplemental movements.

Bodybuilders like Ronnie Coleman and Johnny Jackson and Stan Efferding were insanely strong, despite being the best of a group that is often referred to as 'all show and no go'. You can say it was in spite of being in a sport that didn't prioritize strength but I think it was actually because of it.

Kong is a callback to this era of training and the mindset that existed in it. It sets itself apart because it uses strength as a tool, not the end goal, and the argument I'm making is that this will do the most to make you stronger than the time spent obsessing over the minutiae of strength specialization.

Looking at some of these programs from the greats, something stands out on the strength specialization end. There's a lot of barbell work, and it's done with weight increases in mind. The workouts get relatively heavy and progressive overload is mandatory.

Whether you're doing threes or thirteens, if you can do it with more weight this week than last week, you got stronger

On the other hand, you can see that these programs used a number of sets, a variety of exercises and a crazy amount of reps which is just not typically seen in the training books of todays lifters.

The one arena today where you still tend to see more training variety is in strongman. I've often commented on why I think strongman features some of the biggest backs and strongest deadlifts in the world. I believe it's because they compete in a sport that mandates the ability to knock out high reps in very fatigued conditions with very heavy, overloaded movements.

The average power lifter would never consider doing a set of 15 to 20 in a deadlift for reps, especially on something overloaded like a side handle or elevated deadlift. But strongmen *have* to do it, and usually in hour 4 of an 8 hour day. But even that training leaves something to be desired because of the maximal effort, 'one-and-done' mentality many strongman take; when you leave it all out on the floor during a minute-long deadlift marathon, you aren't typically keen to repeat the effort anytime soon.

Strongmen have to be able to balance the stress of something so taxing as a 15 rep deadlift or squat with their log presses, their keg carries, their stone loads and their yoke walks. So jacking the volume up by using a lot of repeating sets with these compound movements in this threshold would be more detrimental than anything.

But for guys like Kazmaier, who developed insane levels of size and strength before having to dedicate time to specializing in strongman, repeating sets of high-rep barbell movements was par for the course.

Consider all of the variables that contribute to the growth of size and strength.

- If a movement uses a lot of different muscles, it's thought of as a good developer.
- If it puts you through a long range of motion, it's thought of as a good developer.
- If it's stable and allows you to handle a substantial amount of load without risk of falling over, it's a pretty good developer.
- If it has a skill component, meaning that more practice leads to more efficiency, it's said to be a good developer.
- If it allows you to develop an immense amount of fatigue, both localized in the muscle and systemic over the entire body, then it is a good developer.

However good the squat, bench, deadlift and overhead press are as developmental movements, they are at their best as muscle-builders when done for a lot of work and to a point of high fatigue. You are handicapped in your ability to do this when the reps stay low and the work overly 'strength-specific'.

Now, to anybody who is a hopeful competitor, who sees themself competing at strongman or powerlifting nationals one day, note that this is not a call against specializing in every scenario. The whole concept of a periodized routine is to give direction to your training so that you can appropriately balance periods of specialization needed to peak your performance against with dedicated periods of muscle building, like we are talking about here.

One phase widens the base, the other sharpens the tip and neither are optional.

This is a call to acknowledging that specialization has its greatest value when you are minutes away from a big event or contest and has very little value when you are further out.

A soccer player benefits greatly from doing weight training in the off season, but hitting a deadlift PR two weeks before the finals doesn't mean a thing to their game-day performance. Timing is the important factor, here. You always go less specific to more specific, broad to narrow.

TENET #1 - WEAK POINTS FIRST

Kong is written with the first four weeks as an introductory block. The purpose of this block is to build some capacity to get your feet wet so that you actually have some momentum by the time you start incorporating heavy sets with a barbell. It's very common for lifters to start with all of their favorite exercises or all of their contest specific movements in one go, and then burn themselves out too early before they've gotten very far in the progression.

By giving yourself a few weeks to adapt to higher rep ranges and shorter rest periods *first*, you're going to prevent the psychological breakdown that comes with watching your numbers tank. This is really important because training in these thresholds takes some adapting to, and if you have the bad habit of taking your a ball and going home every time you aren't as strong in a workout as you'd like to be, you're never going to get any meaningful work done.

It would be like if a marathoner stopped running every time they were tired.

So the heavy stuff takes a backseat and the smaller stuff goes to the front.

The psychological component, while extremely relevant to most of you, is not the only reason for this first introductory block. The big motivation for putting your weak points first is that it guarantees that you won't skip them.

For instance, say that you've been bench pressing for several years and your numbers have gone steadily up but you've ran into a wall and you haven't really progressed in the last eight months. You look around the gym and notice that your arms are relatively small compared to the other guys in your strength bracket. You might think that if your tricep growth kept pace with your pecs and shoulders, that your bench pressing potential would increase and potentially get you out of this rut.

I would tell you that that's a very reasonable assessment.

Now what many lifters do is they try to outsmart the methods that have worked for the better part of a century. They try to incorporate exotic movement variations, endless specialty bars and convoluted setups that require a team of people holding a fishing scale in order to accurately measure band tension.

Many lifters will do absolutely everything under the sun except prioritize more direct, hard, bodybuilding hypertrophy work to bring up their weak areas.

Other lifters might be willing to put the work in but surmise that they should logically do smaller work last, after the big work. Just like you wouldn't perform very well if you ran a 5K before testing your a hundred meter sprint, you similarly aren't going to do well on your heaviest lifts if you fatigue the smaller components first. But done in reverse order with the heavy stuff at the front and the long draining stuff done at the end, you get the best of all worlds, right?

Now, this would be sound reasoning if lifters had the quality of actually finishing the work that was prescribed for them. One of the biggest problems that keeps modern strength athletes weak is their habit of using any excuse to wrap up a training session and call it good.

Are you tired from work, your warmups dragging and you fell 2 reps short on your first working set? Wrap it up and live to fight another day. You'll have it tomorrow.

Are you crushing PRs, as if the weight is voluntarily moving out of your way? Well, that was a big set, son! Call it a full day's work and go celebrate at Chili's with your boys!

Those extra 15 sets of tricep extensions that are supposed to level-up your pea-shooter arms aren't going to do any good if you only do half the work half the time and smaller movements being put at the end of the workout are *always* the first to get skipped.

By putting weak points first in this introductory cycle, we give you a break from the chase of heavyweights while also making sure that the things that are furthest behind actually get enough work so that they can catch up.

We're also easing you into this threshold of high reps with low rest periods, which takes some getting used to. At the end of this, most of you should experience improvements in smaller muscles that typically lag behind the bigger ones: the triceps, the hamstrings, the delts.

If you're the type of lifter that diligently attacks all of your weak point training, then you shouldn't have any issues. But even for you dedicated lifters, these areas will still get a boost by virtue of having been trained first instead of last.

TENET #2 - DENSITY

Density is an often talked about but is often underutilized approach to increasing size, strength, and performance. Density is simply the amount of work you do over time. So if you do five sets of 10 with 65% of your max, the volume and intensity is exactly the same in a scenario where you have one minute rest periods and five minute rest period.

However, the workout with one minute rest periods represents a much bigger stress because the density of work is so much higher. It's actually such an effective metric that there have been successful programs that use density as the primary driver of progress, ahead of weight. Big Beyond Belief was such a program, billed as the 'most effective muscle building program EVER!' (a cringey overstatement to be sure, but it was a solid routine). It worked by progressively stripping away rest from 3 minutes to 2 to 1.5, all while maintaining or even increasing the total amount of work. As a result, capacity increased, muscle sized increased and strength increased.

Now, I'm not so sure that the effects of density-based training are so monumentally better that density should be the the basket you put all your eggs in. But it is something you should keep track of.

Kong emphasizes short rest periods, especially in the first block where you're only starting out with two sets of 15 on each exercise. This doesn't look like much, but if you're not used to these reps with this many exercises, this will be more than enough to light you up.

You don't have to worry about performing with as much weight as possible. Just worry about the fatigue. Hit your set of 15 with an appropriate amount of weight, rest a brief period of time, gauge if you should add or reduce weight and go again. By the time you get through the third, fourth, fifth exercise, you will feel the punch that high rep movements done with short rests can pack.

As you progress to the pyramids in block 2, density is going to go up even further. The pyramid phase starts the workout with barbell movements, and the increased capacity you have from block 1 should allow you to handle much more total volume in much less time than you could before.

If you survive this program, you should find yourself forever looking at other lifters with judment. As they sit on the bench in between sets of squats, eyes glued to their Instagram, milking every second of recovery off the clock, you will wipe the sweat off your forehead, steady your breathing and go again.

TENET #3 - VOLUME

Volumizing is a strategy that I am a huge fan of and I wrote about it extensively in "Base Strength". The basic idea is that how much work you do is a huge driver of growth and a guaranteed method of accelerating that growth is to acclimate to amounts of work you aren't used to doing.

Periodized programs broadly use a pattern of starting with high volume and then decreasing it over time as the weight gets heavier and more strength specific.

That pattern very broadly makes sense. Start with volume that conditions you and sparks hypertrophy. As you gain muscle, you expose that tissue to heavier loads. Now the nervous system adapts and your body can recruit more motor units at once, making the most of this new found muscle.

The problem is that when you start a volume phase, you are typically very, very deconditioned to volume. Whether you're talking about repeating triples of paused squats and deficit deadlifts in a power lifting specific program or the drop sets and forced reps in a traditional bodybuilding split, your first workout of a new high volume cycle is always going to be one of your worst performances.

Now, let's hope that the first workout didn't scare you off by sending you into the bushes, green-faced and puking up the curry that you foolishly had during your lunch break (you *knew* it was squat day). In the event you show up for week 2 and beyond, you should notice that every subsequent workout benefits from rapid increases in capacity; i.e. the workouts get easier. Not only do you recover in between sets faster, spending less time wheezing with your head in your lap, but you also recover in between reps faster. With the big barbell movements, squats, deads, even presses, this equates to more reps per set and a bigger damn training stress per workout.

By volumizing, we get your toe in the water by starting you out with high reps for only a few sets. The focus is then on adding sets as opposed to adding weight and that means that the highest volume workouts are saved for when you are the most conditioned and can do the most work. The volume you handle at the end of a volumizing phase, four weeks in or so, completely trumps the amount of volume that you could potentially handle if you started out with your highest volume workout in week 1.

Now, obviously you can't increase volume indefinitely, so this has to happen in waves. We start small and increase volume week to week until we hit a crescendo at week 4, at which point we have to drop back and build back up.

That's exactly what Kong does. We build mass on your weak areas and increase your capacity in week 1. Then, as volume climbs high enough to merit a reset, we drop back into block 2 and put the compound barbell movements at the forefront again. Now, we begin building up volume again but this time it's with heavier movements where load takes priority over fatigue.

There have certainly been productive programs that have forsaken volume in favor of ball-busting effort over a few sets. But volume is such an easy dial to turn that I don't know why you would want to leave it out of your training. Not being able to manipulate volume robs you of so many different maneuvers that makes simple problem solving in your training incredibly difficult.

It's like giving your queen up in a chess match.

If you acclimate to volume, you're going to be in better shape and you're going to carry more mass, period. You always have the option of scheduling a period of low volume to focus on peaking strength, and you should notice then that the novelty of really heavy weights with more overall recovery combines to give you an incredible surge of strength in a very short period of time.

That period will also detrain you from high volume, so when you begin working it again it will feel like the first time you trained. You will once again be winded and sore and you will once again see rapid growth. Wash, rinse, repeat.

TENET #4 - HIGH REPS WITH COMPOUNDS

I touched on this a bit already when I talked about the nature of strongman as a sport and why I believe that strongmen tend to have the biggest backs and deadlifts in the world. It is because the sport of strongman is unique in its demand. While strongmen do the same basic barbell movements that other strength athletes do, they do them for an entirely different prescription of work.

Yes, they're pushing their one rep max and yes, they're doing typical volume work. But they're also putting in sets of true density sets where they have to deadlift, squat, and press for reps for the duration of 60 or even 90 seconds, as opposed to confining their work to one defined set.

This is essentially a form of rest-pause. You do a couple of reps, take a breath, do a couple of reps, fidget with your belt, grind a single, chalk up, and one more before time expires…. It allows load to be much, much higher for many more reps with much higher density than you would ever find in a traditional working set. In addition to that, long carries with yokes and farmer walk handles, high rep loading events and death medleys represent a ratio of "load-to-effort-to-time" that just simply isn't seen in any other mode of training.

Anybody who transitioned to strongman from typical barbell training knows how hard it is at first to work your deadlifts around the fatigue and soreness you feel from event day. And many have reported seeing their deadlift go up dramatically without any deadlifting; simply by doing farmer picks, stone loads and sandbag carries does the hips and back grow stronger.

Kong was written with the benefits of long, hard sets in mind. You aren't going to be limiting your work with squats, deadlifts presses and rows to 15 seconds or less. Sets are going to last 30, 45 seconds, even a minute.

Even in the last four weeks of Kong, the heaviest phase, you are going to finish your heavy sets with a high rep amrap. By the time you reach the end of this program, sets of 12 and 15 should be as simple as walking up a flight of stairs. You should no longer get sweaty palms at the thought of volume or capacity work and you should be eager to chase new PRs at these rep ranges (which should come easy for some time by virtue of them being new).

We can look to some of the biggest, baddest lifters from eras gone by and evaluate the amount of work that led to their physiques. I mentioned Bill Kazmaier previously, who would squat and deadlift in the same workout for multiple high-rep sets.

Here is his infamous routine:

MONDAY
Bench (heavy) warm-up, then 4 sets x 10 reps
Wide Grip Bench 3 sets x 10 reps
Narrow Grip Bench 3 sets x 10 reps
Front Delt Raise 4 sets x 8 reps
Dumbell Seated Press 4 sets x 10 reps
Side Delt Raise 4 sets x 10 reps
Lying Tricep Push (after 2 warm-up sets) 6 sets x 10 reps
Tricep Push Down 4 sets x 10 reps

TUESDAY

Squat (heavy) warm-up, then 4 sets x 10 reps
Deadlift (light) warm-up, then 3 sets x 10 reps
Shrugs 2 sets x 15-40 reps, 1 set x 10-20 reps
Seated Hammer Curls 4 sets x 12 reps
Standing Curl 4 sets x 10 reps
Close Grip Chin Ups 3 sets x max on each set
Seated Row 4 sets x 10 reps
Leg Extensions 3 sets x 10 reps
Leg Curl 3 sets x 10 reps
Calf Raise 3 sets x 15-25 reps

THURSDAY

Bench (light) warm-up, then 3 sets x 10 reps
Wide Grip Bench 3 sets x 10 reps
Narrow Grip Bench 3 sets x 10 reps
Dumbell Seated Press (heavy) warm-up, then 4 sets x 8 reps
Front Delt Raise 4 sets x 10 reps
Tennis Backhand Cable Extensions 4 sets x 10 reps
Prone Tricep Extension 4 sets x 10 reps

FRIDAY

Deadlift (heavy) warm-up, then 4 sets x 8 reps
Squat (light) warm-up, then 4 sets of x10 reps
Shrugs (heavy) 4 sets x 10-15 reps
Seated Hammer Curl 4 sets x 8 reps
Concentration Curl 4 sets x 12 reps
One Arm Row – 3 positions 3 sets x 10 reps
Wide Grip Pull (down to chest) 4 sets x 10 reps
Leg Extensions 3 sets x 10 reps
Leg Curl 3 sets x 10 reps
Calf Raise 3 sets x 15-25 reps

Roger Estep, who was photographed in one of the most iconic powerlifting pictures ever taken, was known for lifting immense weights while looking like an in-season bodybuiler. He wrote the 3-day per week program below specifically for new powerlifters:

Leg Raise– 50 / **Crunch–** 50 / **Jackknife–** 50

Squat– Two warmup sets (15 reps and 8 reps). Work sets: 3 x 8, then add weight and do 2 x 5

Bench Press– Two warmup sets (15 reps and 8 reps). Work sets: 3 x 8, then add weight and do 2 x 5

Seated DB Curl– 3 x 8

Incline Tricep Extension– 3 x 8

Deadlift– Two warmup sets (15 reps and 8 reps). Work sets: 3 x 8, then add weight and do 2 x 5

DB Row– 3 x 8

Behind the Neck Press– 3 x 8

Shrugs– 4 x 6

Calf Raise– 3 x 12

As Jamie Lewis from "Plague of Strength" commented in regards to Roger's program:

> "The following is a... beginner program for powerlifters, which you might be interested to find contains a sh**load of bodybuilding, because prior to the invention of the internet, powerlifters weren't drooling fucking r**ards who feared hard work more than rich college girls fear work of any kind. This sh** might not blow your socks off, but it might be of interest in that it involves more than just the big three lifts, which is nigh on f**king heresy at this point with new jack lifters."

The man has a way with words. But he ain't wrong.

The average person looks at that and immediately thinks over training and I say, nay. If you give yourself time to adapt and progress at a reasonable rate and if you eat like you're actually in danger of going up a weight class, you will be absolutely astonished at how fast your body grows to keep up.

TENET #5 - FATIGUED STRENGTH

This one is going to be completely new to most of you.

It's true that if you go into a heavy set of work fatigued, the amount of weight you use isn't going to be as high. You are going to be fighting against other limitations besides your nervous system and how efficiently it operates and that means the work will not be exactly 'strength-specific'.

That does not mean you don't get stronger.

Remember, Kong is anti-specialization. The time for peaking strength by prioritizing neurological development at the expense of everything else will come in the future with some other program and, when it does, it will be the icing on the cake. For now, you want to condition yourself to be able to hang, to be able to put out repeated bouts of effort as fatigue continues to build through the course of a workout.

This requires training and practice. It takes time for you to adapt to this type of work.

Remembering that we are here to train and not to test, that our job is to grow and not just prove to ourselves that we could lift what we did last week, we are going to be doing heavy work *after* we are already fatigued from the sets that came before.

Heresy, I know.

This is going to happen in phase one when you try your hand at pressing movements after your triceps are already blown or when you schedule squats and deadlifts after copious amounts of direct hamstring work. This is also going to happen in phase 2, when we move into pyramids and we work up to heavy sets of five *after* doing challenging sets of 12, 10, 8 reps. The weight you're going to be reaching for these heaviest sets is going to pale in comparison to what you would do fresh, and that is absolutely okay. In fact, that's ideal.

If you handle the same weight at the end of a pyramid that you would if you did that set first as a top set, I'm going to tell you that those first sets were not pushed hard enough and the training stimulus is going to suffer as a result. Look at all sets as being created equal in this program and strain on the 12s the way you would on the 3s.

There are a handful of benefits to doing this. One is the obvious increase in training stress that you sustain from the continously high fatigue through the entire workout. The strain starts from set one and it only gets worse from there.

But the other is that your general capacity is going to absolutely skyrocket. No more will you be the person that has to give yourself 20 minutes to warm up in order to get right for your first squat or deadlift sets. This is, importantly, I think, a sign that you're in adequate shape, that you might actually be deadly in other arenas that benefit from strength as opposed to only being strong when the conditions are perfect.

A sufficiently conditioned lifter should be able to knock off the number of warmup sets they need to be 'ready' with 30 seconds to a minute in between and, if needed, be ready to handle their top working weight within five minutes or less. This is a HUGE advantage when you compete, as most lifters train themselves to be tempermental and to fall apart when conditions are volatile.

Powerlifters often botch their attempts because they can't pace their warmups appropriately. And, God helped me, let's not forget the 'competitors' that cite fatigue from the long meet day as the cause of their failed final deadlift attempt. If nine reps over a 10 hour day causes you to lose dramatic amounts of strength then, brother, you need to go back to the drawing board.

This is extremely relevant in strongman, where warm ups are basically non-existent. Nationals routinely features 400+ athletes with just 5 lanes worth of equipment: that means that 400 people have the designated 30 minutes or so to warm up on 5 pieces of equipment. That's especially egregious for a sport that revolves around testing a lifter's ability to move insane loads in a highly fatigued state. Not surprisingly, it doesn't workout well for those who aren't conditioned or adaptable.

So, by actually dedicating time to building a motor so that you can recover quickly in between sets, you're going to get exponentially more out of your training. And on meet day, while everybody else is slowing down, you can take satisfaction in knowing that you're just getting started.

If you're familiar with any of the other books I've written on programming, you know that there are some things to watch out for in any given strength program. The big thing that we worry about when our priority is strength-specific (i.e. hitting the biggest possible numbers) is recovery. Lack of it is one of the biggest problem that lifters run into early on when they think the secret is just "more, more, more".

In the beginning, you might be able to sustain a certain rate of progress by just going harder each time. This is especially true when you're not very strong. Counterintuitively, less developed lifters can actually train harder and more frequently than those who are stronger, more experienced and more conditioned. The basic idea is that newbies are not trained or conditioned enough to generate enough stress to cause a substantial disruption to their body.

Even though your muscles grow to adapt, all of the other structures in your body also have to handle the trauma caused by your heavy squats, deadlifts and presses, and the fact is that 800 pounds just causes a lot more damage than 300. While you might increase the amount of muscle you have 5 fold over the course of your training lifetime, you aren't going to see that growth in your adrenal glands. So stronger lifters would do well to keep in mind that a smaller dose *tends* to goes a longer way.

They also have to keep in mind that there are certain demonstrations of effort that, while once essential for progress, will now prolong the amount of time it takes to get back at full strength again.

Here's an example: if you bench press for a few easy sets of six you might be able to clock enough volume to grow but the stress that you suffered might not be so high as to require very much recovery.

Now, if instead of that you decided to go and swing for the fences and grinded through set after set of some of the hardest triples you've ever done in your life, you might notice that your next workout is worse, not better. After a full week of recovery, you would come into the gym eager to get after it only to find the bar moves like crap. You aren't sore, you feel 100% but you still have to drop 10% off of your typical working weight just to get through the workout.

This is the most easily prevented problem that lifters will run into, causing years of stagnation and frustration before it's realized that they need to stop bashing their head against the wall and commit to a comprehensive training plan that at least tries to account for recovery.

To be able to predict your performance workout to workout, you have to know what causes your strength to suffer and it's different for each lift. Benching usually recovers a bit quicker and something like deadlifting usually takes much longer. The best squatters and deadlifters in the world will often hit their heaviest squat attempt three or even four weeks out from their meet date and take the rest of the time to taper down the amount of work, allowing their body to recover in the process.

The biggest hits to the nervous system happen on really hard efforts with big lifts, especially ones that use a lot of weight over a long range of motion. One of the benefits of Kong is the prescription of weak points first in block 1 and focusing on fatigued strength with higher reps in block 2. We don't have to worry about the CNS getting smoked because the thresholds we are working in are not laser focused on it. That's the benefit of taking time from very strength specific work; the nervous system isn't the primary structure being taxed so we can cut loose and push a bit harder.

When you're doing sets of 12, 10, 8, when you're doing the repeating sets every week and volumizing the whole way, the only thing you have to worry about recovery-wise is that you aren't so brutally sore that you can't do the next workout scheduled and that your joints and connective tissue can handle the amount of work without you developing an overuse issue.

Of course, both of those things are at play in any program you will ever run. It's the fact of not having to tiptoe around your nervous system recovery that is the huge win here. Just focus on cranking effort over the weeks and meeting the prescription for each workout and you will adapt.

TENET #6 - LOAD VARIATION

Y ou have a lot of options of how to arrange the sets and reps in any given program. The easiest way to plan them out is through sets across (i.e. 4x5, where all sets and reps are the same).

Sometimes these are done for ascending weight, meaning the weight goes up until you hit a top set at that rep range. Very often, it's implied that the weight is being kept static throughout the entire workout.

While that works very well and some of the exercises in this program even feature sets across, Kong leans heavily on load variation as a way of exposing you to a variety of training thresholds.

By pyramiding up and down and changing the weight and the rep range set to set, a greater variety of muscle fibers are stimulated, a greater variety of energy systems are taxed and an element of novelty is added to your training that should renew your interest in your workout and keep you engaged.

One of the most notorious applications of the implementation of load variation is in the programs of Boris Sheiko. If you have ran a program from the GOAT of powerlifting coaches, you know how each workout involves a continuous change in weight from set to set, often times pyramiding up and back down, sometimes even mixing up the sets and changing weights in a seemingly sporadic and random fashion. For the competitive movements that make up 90% of the program, no adjacent sets are ever the same.

The idea is that changing the weights interrupts your anticipation of what the following set is going to be like. Yes, you get the varied stimulus of all of the different sets, but you also stay focused longer, are more eager to get through each set and you subsequently get a better result from the entire session.

Monotony is a killer in training. If you can squeeze a little more enthusiasm from each set by doing something as simple as changing the weights, you can add quite a bit of 'oomph' to your training.

TENET #7 - PHASE POTENTIATION

Phase potentiation is the arrangement of training blocks in a logical order, where each block of training 'potentiates', or increases your potential for, the following phase. This is extremely important in most sports because there are so many variables to balance and timing is crucial.

Think of the general type of training that any athlete does in the off season. The closer they get to their meet, the less important that training becomes and the more important their handling of actual game day scenarios is. Any martial artist should be lifting weights, doing cardio, and building a basic athletic base in the off season but two weeks before a big match, they shouldn't be doing much else that isn't mimicking the actual fight.

With strength, we always put muscle growth first in the macrocycle. If we increase the amount of muscle we have, we can then do strength specific work afterwards that focuses on your neurological recruitment of that muscle mass. So we build up a lot of raw materials first and then we focus on making better use of those raw materials.

It's a very logical pattern to do things, especially when you're getting ready for a meet.

Kong utilizes phase potentiation by exposing you to training that is useful for size and capacity and then applying that new size and capacity to blocks of training that make new use of them.

The first phase has a lot of isolation movements, a lot of machines and unilateral work. It has smaller movements done for a lot of reps and the amount of volume increases session to session. By the time you get to week four, you should have a bit more muscle to show for your effort, fewer weak points and better conditioning. This gets your toe in the water and sets you up for block two, which starts each workout with pyramids with the heavier compound movements that we initially had at the back of the line.

Going into block three, we flip that on its head. The pyramids now become reverse pyramid, where we are finally prioritizing moving the most weight when we are the most fresh. After the top set at the start of the workout, we then drop the weight and move to high rep sets, utilizing post activation potentiation to get more out of thm.

With phase potentiation, the changes we make phase to phase compound the growth stimulus and the end result is you leave this program a lot bigger, stronger and more capable than when you started.

PROGRAM BREAKDOWN

KONG is broken up into 3 blocks, each of which increases volume and weight over their 4-week period.

RPE

This is an 'RPE' based program (which, virtually most hypertrophy or bodybuilding inspired workouts are). Now, some of you might be used to gauging RPE for your singles, triples and sets of five. But doing it for sets of 12, 15 or 20 is an entirely different ball game. It's not quite going to line up with the normal instruction of associating RPE with reps in reserve; such as RPE 9 being equal to 1 good rep left in the tank, RPE 7 meaning 3 reps left, etc.

You're going to have to find a more general approach to gauging RPE because high reps come with a lot more variables than singles and doubles. This range of work increases fatigue and pain substantially and with very high reps, the difference between 3 and 5 reps in reserve is negligible. You will also be relying on different energy systems with different movements; sets of 15 on bench will create a lot of local muscular fatigue but the same work on lunges and RDLs will feel cardiovascular.

So if you are pushing through sets of 20 on leg presses and your legs are on fire and nausea is creeping up your stomach with each rep, that might account for a higher RPE then the simple calculation of how many more reps you could do with a gun pointed towards your head.

You are also going to have to get good at anticipating how fatigued one set is going to leave you for the next one. You might finish a set of 15 with a few in the tank and think, "I feel pretty damn good, I'm going to keep the weight the same", only to get halfway through the next set and realize that you've already blown your RPE wad.

I can't stress this enough: having this type of insight into how your body responds to the stress of an individual set is a minimum requirement for being considered a lifter. It's like being able to parallel park in order to get your license; it ain't optional.

But don't stress; you don't need to walk a tightrope in finding an exact RPE on this program. The spirit of the RPE progression is that each block starts off relatively easy and gets harder week-to-week. Since the reps either stay the same or decrease over each block, it's implied that RPE increases by increasing weight.

So choose weights in week one of each block that leave some damn room for improvement. Virtually none of you reading this are going to be conditioned to this many sets of 15 and 20 in the first week (especially on leg day) so you have a big margin for error. I recommend undershooting on week 1 and overshooting on week 4. Even if you go a bit to light in week 1 you will still likely be very sore and you'll get some insight as to how to accurately gauge effort in the context a of crazier hypertrophy rep ranges.

BLOCK 1

The first block is the introductory block. This is essentially a body building split that focuses on muscle groups as opposed to movement patterns. This is going to be a welcome change for most of you that are used to only orienting your workouts around barbell movements.

Many of the muscles are trained twice per week with the ones that tend to get hit the hardest with the big lifts being used for less frequency.

> Day 1 - triceps, delts, and pecs
> Day 2 - hams, glutes and quads
> Day 3 - back, delts and bis
> Day 4 - quads, hams and glutes
> Day 5 - bis, back and tris

You'll notice that the order of the exercises gets jumbled session to session; muscle groups that lead on one day might be done towards the end on another day. This ensures that everything gets hit with high frequency while also having a day to be done when you are absolutely fresh.

For progressive overload, the program follows a simple volumizing approach.

The first week, most everything is done for two sets of 15, with a few exercises done for 20 and a few exercises done for 12. This is all done at RPE 7, which means somewhat challenging but still considerably short of failure. Now, this is going to be the hardest thing for you guys to gauge because RPE generally denotes how many reps are left in the tank. That's a very different sensation at 15 reps than it is at 3 reps.

The point is you shouldn't be within more than three reps of failure on your first exercise and likely further away than that. And based on how fatigued you are, you might actually need to drop the weight slightly going into the second. Every workout, you should notice improvements in your ability to sustain effort for those reps.

Week 2 jumps to 3 sets on everything, cranking the volume up by 50%. Week 3 moves some exercises to 4 sets and week four drops the reps, allowing you to get quite a bit heavier.

For rest periods, I recommend trying to keep it to a minute rest in between exercises. You can take a longer break between exercises further down through the workout if you're starting to struggle. This density component is an absolutely huge component to making progress in this program.

BLOCK 2

Block 2 starts to sneak in strength-specificity by putting compound barbell movements front and center again. After 4 weeks of doing smaller isolation work first, now you get to get under a barbell and throw some weight around.

All of the main movements are starting with a traditional pyramid: 12, 10, 8, 5, 12.

The main movements are all disadvantaged developmental movements; that is, movements that go through a wider range of motion and don't allow as much weight to be used. The list is seated presses, stiff leg deadlifts, strict bent rows, close grip benches and high bar squats.

The reps move forward as the program gets heavier, moving from fives to threes and from eights to sixes. The RPE goes up week to week, again, implying that more weight should be used.

Notice as you get better at selecting weights, how much the overall training stress increases. Yes, you can get very fatigued just by going hard, but if you can hold back just enough effort to handle more weight across all of these sets and reps, that represents a bigger total mathematical stress from the volume.

BLOCK 3

Block 3 maintains the same split as block 2 but swaps the main exercises for more overloaded variations.

> Strict presses go to push presses.
> Stiff leg deadlifts go to 13 inch deadlifts.
> Strict barbell rows go to Pendlay rows.
> Close grip bench goes to wide grip bench.
> Close stance squat goes to wide stance squat.

The pyramids for the main movements are now reverse pyramids, which means you are starting with your heaviest top set when you are fresh. The extra load from not being fatigued combined with the weight you can handle on these advantaged variations should result in a HUGE shift in stress.

Block 3 is where you should be like a dog on a leash, ready to be cut loose.

You should feel like you have a second gear going into this top set because you don't have all of the fatigue built up that you had in each day of the prior 8 weeks.

There is a bit of a learning curve with these exercises. Many of you might take a week or two to get really comfortable with these movements if you haven't done them before. Just take as many warmup sets as you need to feel comfortable and stay true to the RPE.

This is the block that you should be thinking of throughout this entire program. You should be excited to get in here and throw some weight around. Also, take the back off sets seriously; at this point, finishing an exercise with a set of 15 or 12 should be like walking up a flight of stairs, so use your newly acquired motor and go for blood.

This block is still a lot of volume, a lot more than many strength athletes handle on a regular basis, and it is still the lowest volume part of the entire program. It should go without saying that, after molding yourself to the demands of this program, the way you approach training should never quite be the same.

KONG

BLOCK 1

Day 1	Week 1 (RPE 7)	Week 2 (RPE 5, 7, 10)	Week 3 (RPE 5, 7, 10)	Week 4 (RPE 5, 7, 10, 10)
JM Press	2x15	3x12	4x12	4x10
French Press	2x15	3x12	3x12	3x10
V-Handle Pressdown	2x20	3x15	3x15	3x12
Front Raise w/ DBs	2x15	3x12	4x12	4x10
Upright Row	2x15	3x12	3x12	3x10
Barbell Incline Bench	2x15	3x12	3x12	3x10
Machine Chest Press	2x15	3x12	3x12	3x10
Cable Crossover	2x20	3x15	3x15	3x12

Chest pressing work done after tricep and shoulder work is going to be different for you. Your triceps and deltoids are going to be shockingly more fatigued than you're used to because you've likely never led a workout with those muscles. This should be an eye opening experience as to the amount and type of fatigue that causes rapid muscle growth.

You're going to feel exceptionally weak movements like barbell benching, The weight is going to have to drop substantially from what you are used to. Don't use that as an excuse to skip the work or treat it as unimportant. In the next few weeks you will condition to this amount of work and you will be closer to ranges that you're used to training in. But how much improvement you see by the end depends on how you handle these early session so take them seriously.

Day 2	Week 1 (RPE 7)	Week 2 (RPE 5, 7, 10)	Week 3 (RPE 5, 7, 10)	Week 4 (RPE 5, 7, 10, 10)
Hamstring Curl	2x20	3x15	3x15	3x12
Romanian Deadlift	2x15	3x12	4x12	4x10
Leg Press	2x15	3x12	3x12	3x10
Walking Lunge w/ DBs	2x12 each	3x12 each	3x12 each	3x10 each
Leg Extension	2x15	3x12	3x12	3x10

Hamstring curls into Romanian deadlifts into leg presses into lunges is another combination that is going to throw you for a loop. Even if you keep the weight very light on the few sets of hamstring curl,s the little bit of blood flow into that area is going to make the Romanian deadlifts burn like hell.

This one tweak of putting the hamstring work before the knee dominant movements usually leads to extreme soreness in the posterior chain. The beauty of this is that you're likely to be inclined to sandbag the weight with these high rep lower body movements the first week anyways but that actually works to your benefit because the soreness is usually crippling.

But don't get too unambitious because, by weeks 3 and 4 you should be putting out a lot of effort on those RPE 10 work sets all the way through to the last exercise.

Day 3	Week 1 (RPE 7)	Week 2 (RPE 5, 7, 10)	Week 3 (RPE 5, 7, 10)	Week 4 (RPE 5, 7, 10, 10)
Behind the Neck Press	2x15	3x12	4x12	4x10
One Arm Lateral	2x15	3x12	3x12	3x10
One Arm DB Row	2x20	3x15	3x15	3x12
Lat Pulldown	2x15	3x12	4x12	4x10
Hammer Curl	2x15	3x12	3x12	3x10
Barbell Curl 21s	2 sets	3 sets	3 sets	3 sets

I'm a huge fan of behind the neck presses as a developmental movement, provided it doesn't aggravate some pre-existing shoulder issue. These high reps should be a good opportunity to get the movement down and coax some mobility and durability in that area. Treat it like a Jefferson curl or any other movement that puts you in a vulnerable position with the aim of making you bulletproof there.

For the lateral raises and dumbbell rows, I like to prescribe a good amount of body English over super strictt reps; how much you use is up to you. The big trade-off is whether you're going to use more aggression, speed and weight or if you are going to use tempo and control with a lighter weights to keep the stress high. One isn't necessarily better than the other, they are just different. As long as you aren't flopping around like an epileptic trout, either approach will lead to growth.

The 21s are there because, well, I was feeling sentimental. This is everybody's first introduction into advanced fatigue techniques that create more of a crippling burn in the target muscle than straight sets and reps can do by themselves.

I love 21s for hammering weak areas and I threw them in here for biceps because it was just an efficient way to hit a smaller muscle that likely isn't the biggest priority for most of you. But I've done 21s with hamstrings, with shoulders, with quads, even with compound movements.

In a future installment I could easily dedicate a lot of text to these types of techniques, like using limited range of motion to keep tension on the muscle or executing a short double-pump at the end range of motion to trap blood and reach deeper levels of fatigue. There's a lot of fun to be had with those types of things and you are more than welcome to experiment with them on the smaller movements here.

Remember this is a hypertrophy program so we put a high premium on creating a huge amount of fatigue directly in the belly of the muscle. The very highreps will get most of you there. But as time goes on and you adapt (and you will be a lot bigger by the time you do) you'll have to get creative.

Day 4	Week 1 (RPE 7)	Week 2 (RPE 5, 7, 10)	Week 3 (RPE 5, 7, 10)	Week 4 (RPE 5, 7, 10, 10)
Leg Extension	2x20	3x15	3x15	3x12
Squat	2x15	3x12	4x12	4x10
Weighted Back Extension	2x15	3x12	3x12	3x10
Single Leg Press	2x15	3x12	3x12	3x10
Hamstring Curl	2x15	3x12	4x12	4x10

The second lower body workout now starts with quads instead of hamstrings, which should be a blessing because most of you are probably suffering from a swollen posterior right about now. This is far from a reprieve, though.

Just like with the hamstring work coming first on Day 2, doing leg extensions and trapping a little bit of blood in the quads is enough to make the squats much much more strenuous for the same weight and effort. Once again, you will be sore from this. With the squat, resist the urge to chase what you think should be a competitive number for a 15 repper. This isn't Super Squats style breathing squats; not that that is an effective method, it certainly is. But putting that type of intensity into this type of program is going to send most of you to the bushes and eliminate any chance you had of actually finishing the workout.

Again, start conservatively, get comfortable with finishing the workout and then add weight where you can. I don't care if you need to drop to 10% of your max to get through all of the Reps; it's up to you to pick an appropriate weight.

Day 5	Week 1 (RPE 7)	Week 2 (RPE 5, 7, 10)	Week 3 (RPE 5, 7, 10)	Week 4 (RPE 5, 7, 10, 10)
Barbell Curl	2x15	3x12	4x12	4x10
Alternating DB Curl	2x15	3x12	3x12	3x10
Concentration Curl	2x15	3x12	3x12	3x10
Cable Row	2x15	3x12	3x12	3x10
Machine High Row	2x15	3x12	3x12	3x10
Dips	2x15	3x12	4x12	4x10
Rope Pressdown	2x20	3x15	3x15	3x12

This is a pure vanity workout and the session that many of you can look forward to seeing the biggest improvements in over the first block. It's extremely common these days for strength-oriented trainees to minimize the importance of things like bicep or direct back and tricep work, so when you do finally commit to putting them front and center, they usually go off like gangbusters.

After the maassacre you survived in the form of the previous two lower body workouts, this is going to feel like a bit of a vacation. Go in relaxed and ready to enjoy yourself; these are the sessions that are fun and give immediate gratification while still adding something to your training long-term.

For the alternating dumbbell curls, try to keep your palms up in both arms through the entire set. For the dips, use as much band assistance as you need to get the reps in the right rpe range. If this is to complicated or isn't an option you can simply just do the two sets to failure, using a bench dip if parallel bar dips are too hard. For you smaller guys with strong upper bodies, feel free to add a little bit of weight or to wrap a band from the handles to around your neck if two sets of 15 with your body weight is child's play.

It's very likely that many of you won't have access to specific exercises mentioned here and that's perfectly okay. Some of these are movements that I really like and others are just variation for the sake of variation. It's not that anyone movement is magical or essential but each one checks a box in a program that leans on having a lot of variety. So don't stress out about swapping a machine or cable movement for a free weight equivalent based on whatever is available to you.

BLOCK 2

Day 1	Week 5 (RPE 7)	Week 6 (RPE 8)	Week 7 (RPE 8)	Week 8 (RPE 9)
Seated Military Press	12, 10, 8, 5, 12	10, 8, 5, 3, 12	10, 8, 5, 3, 8, 12	8, 5, 3, 5, 8, 12
DB Shoulder Press	12, 10, 8	12, 10, 8	10, 8, 6, 12	10, 8, 6, 12
DB Lateral Raise	12, 10, 8	12, 10, 8	10, 8, 6, 12	10, 8, 6, 12
Dips	12, 10, 8	12, 10, 8	10, 8, 6, 12	10, 8, 6, 12
Skull Crusher	12, 10, 8	12, 10, 8	10, 8, 6, 12	10, 8, 6, 12
V-Bar Pressdown	12, 10, 8	12, 10, 8	10, 8, 6, 12	10, 8, 6, 12

So, you made it through the high rep, volumizing, bodybuilding hell. Congratulations. Even if you feel like you're static lifts took a dump, you should notice some tangible size increases in your arms, shoulders, back and legs and your conditioning should be through the effing roof. We are going to use both of those things and apply them back toAre compound movements and we should be able to leverage those improvements to do more volume and build more fatigued with them than we were ever able to do before.

We're using pyramids now and the rpes should be used to roughly estimate effort on each set. That means the sets of 12 10 and 8 are not passive warm-ups going into a table set of 5 or 3. They are working sets. Treat them as such. This is where we engage enough fatigue strength work that I mentioned as part of 10 it number five. Again your table sets might seem meager compared to what you can do fresh but we are here to train not test what you can do fresh. You will see that number pick up closer to what a fresh performance would look like as you adapt to this and not to sign that you've gotten bigger more conditioned and a hell of a lot stronger.

I like seated military presses as our main developer here, but if there isn't a rack were reasonably simple setup available you can certainly do them standing.

For the dips, you would ideally be using extra weight and increasing to meet the lower wraps down the pyramid like you would with any other exercise. But the fatigue that's going to build up in the first part of this workout is going to make many of you lucky to be able to use your body weight. So do your best to fit the rep ranges with whatever assistance or resistance method you have available but do not stress being exact here. Just like with block one, if you have to settle for bench dips because regular dips are too hard, that's fine and if you have to settle for work with the same weight because you are limited in your ability to precisely scale the weight set to set, that's fine too. For this movement, we can be satisfied with 3 to 4 challenging working sets at any rep count close to the prescribed number.

Day 2	Week 5 (RPE 7)	Week 6 (RPE 8)	Week 7 (RPE 8)	Week 8 (RPE 9)
Stiff Leg Deadlifts	12, 10, 8, 5, 12	10, 8, 5, 3, 12	10, 8, 5, 3, 8, 12	8, 5, 3, 5, 8, 12
Weighted Back Extension	12, 10, 8	12, 10, 8	10, 8, 6, 12	10, 8, 6, 12
Leg Extension	12, 10, 8	12, 10, 8	10, 8, 6, 12	10, 8, 6, 12
Bulgarian Split Squat	12, 10, 8	12, 10, 8	10, 8, 6, 12	10, 8, 6, 12
Leg Press	12, 10, 8	12, 10, 8	10, 8, 6, 12	10, 8, 6, 12
Hamstring Curl	12, 10, 8	12, 10, 8	10, 8, 6, 12	10, 8, 6, 12

Hallelujah, we are doing are deadlifts first! This is an opportunity that is not to be wasted. You should be super eager to demonstrate some strength on the stiff leg deadlifts given that you are doing them fresh. In fact, you should feel like you have an extra gear since your hamstrings aren't already sagging with pooled blood by the time you're walking up to the barbell.

Stiff-legged deadlift differ from Romanian deadlifts in a few subtle ways. Firstly, I want you going to the ground each time instead of floating the weight at the bottom, as you do in an RDL. Second, posture takes a back seat. That doesn't mean that you let your back fold like a wet piece of cardboard but, in order to keep your knees back and hips high and have the bar start on the ground, it's acceptable to have just a bit of given your back. As long as you are bracing hard through your midsection and putting the movement in your hips, you will be A-okay.

For the weighted back extensions, just about every one of you should be using weight. I find myself having to yell at people over this more than anything else because, for some reason, people think a few sets of bodyweight back extensions is going to do the magical trick in building a strong posterior. Most sedentary mother's I know can do a set of back extensions with a 25lb plate. Don't skip out here.

For the Bulgarian split squats, stand next to a rack or post that you can grab onto with one arm to balance and hold a dumbbell with the other. This will make it much easier to get through the working sets, especially as you fatigue from the early work.

And for the leg presses just go hard as you effing can.

Day 3	Week 5 (RPE 7)	Week 6 (RPE 8)	Week 7 (RPE 8)	Week 8 (RPE 9)
Bent Barbell Row	12, 10, 8, 5, 12	10, 8, 5, 3, 12	10, 8, 5, 3, 8, 12	8, 5, 3, 5, 8, 12
Wide Grip Cable Row	12, 10, 8	12, 10, 8	10, 8, 6, 12	10, 8, 6, 12
One Arm Lat Pulldown	12, 10, 8	12, 10, 8	10, 8, 6, 12	10, 8, 6, 12
DB Pullover	12, 10, 8	12, 10, 8	10, 8, 6, 12	10, 8, 6, 12
Preacher Curl	12, 10, 8	12, 10, 8	10, 8, 6, 12	10, 8, 6, 12
Alternating DB Curl	12, 10, 8	12, 10, 8	10, 8, 6, 12	10, 8, 6, 12
Cable Curl	12, 10, 8	12, 10, 8	10, 8, 6, 12	10, 8, 6, 12

Good old-fashioned bent barbell rows are the main movement for this primary upper back day. They will follow the same pyramid progression that your squats, presses and deadlifts do in this block. Everything else here is pretty self-explanatory, although the dumbbell pullovers might be a little bit new to some of you. This is one of those movements to get phased in and out generationally that I expect to be popular at some arbitrary point in the future just because people remembered, "Oh yeah, that's a thing people used to do to get big and strong".

Just position yourself perpendicular on a flat bench as if you were about to do a set of glute barbell bridges. with a diamond grip, hold a single dumbbell above your chest keep your elbows slightly bent and let the dumbbell arc back behind your head. Stretch as far as you comfortably can without any shoulder issues. This provides a pretty big stretch through the rib cage (in fact, it was thought to be a method of expanding your rib cage) and it also does some good work for the lats and pecs. Not much of a primary builder by itself, it's still a valuable exercise, especially at the back end of a s*** ton of volume.

Again, for any exercises that require pieces of equipment that you don't have access to, like a preacher bench, any substitute you come up with for that muscle group will suffice.

Day 4	Week 5 (RPE 7)	Week 6 (RPE 8)	Week 7 (RPE 8)	Week 8 (RPE 9)
Close Grip Bench Press	12, 10, 8, 5, 12	10, 8, 5, 3, 12	10, 8, 5, 3, 8, 12	8, 5, 3, 5, 8, 12
Wide Grip Incline Bench Press	12, 10, 8	12, 10, 8	10, 8, 6, 12	10, 8, 6, 12
Machine Chest Press	12, 10, 8	12, 10, 8	10, 8, 6, 12	10, 8, 6, 12
DB Fly	12, 10, 8	12, 10, 8	10, 8, 6, 12	10, 8, 6, 12
Seated Dip Machine	12, 10, 8	12, 10, 8	10, 8, 6, 12	10, 8, 6, 12

Day 4	Week 5 (RPE 7)	Week 6 (RPE 8)	Week 7 (RPE 8)	Week 8 (RPE 9)
Close Grip Bench Press	12, 10, 8, 5, 12	10, 8, 5, 3, 12	10, 8, 5, 3, 8, 12	8, 5, 3, 5, 8, 12
2 Hand Overhead Tricep Extension	12, 10, 8	12, 10, 8	10, 8, 6, 12	10, 8, 6, 12

Close-grip bench is one of my favorite disadvantaged pressing movements. Regular competitive style pressing typically over-builds the muscles that move at the shoulder, like the pecs and delts, but don't typically cause phenomenal growth in the extremities. Well, elite pressing, I would argue, mandates elite arm development as much as it mandates anything else. By moving more through the elbow joint, we get stronger in the elbows and that leads to strength that is going to carry you through in anything that looks like a pressing movement.

Don't go super close on your grip, we don't want wrist flexibility to be the limiting factor here. I like to go thumbless because I feel like it placees more stress in my elbow/tricep but that is a personal preference. I also like to stop an inch or so off my chest as I find the getting all the way down usually creates a bunch of awkward discomfort in my joints and doesn't really add anything to the exercise. Again personal preference.

Don't overthink it, we aren't doing surgery here. The point is that you are doing a pressing movement that is in a mildly more disadvantaged position than what you are used to. Doing it long enough to get better at it is all you need to grow.

With barbell pressing movements, I like to demonstrate control. I conceptualize it like I'm developing mastery of a basic movement so that I can be worth a damn what I'm on the platform on meet day. I think of it like a martial artist practicing Tai Chi. The more dominance I have over the weights in phases like these the more confident I am that I can be aggressive and violent in heavier phases.

Machines, however, don't have a skill component and serve as a instrument of blunt force trauma to the muscles being used. For them, I take a different approach. I tend to limit range of motion here usually operating in the middle range and I don't rest at all between reps. Cycling through reps quicker create a substrate deficit faster and creates a deeper level of fatigue.

But that's all personal preference. Play around but don't treat any one method like it's the difference between you growing and not. It isn't.

One more time: for equipment you don't have, swap exercises as needed.

Day 5	Week 5 (RPE 7)	Week 6 (RPE 8)	Week 7 (RPE 8)	Week 8 (RPE 9)
High Bar Close Stance Squat	12, 10, 8, 5, 12	10, 8, 5, 3, 12	10, 8, 5, 3, 8, 12	8, 5, 3, 5, 8, 12
Machine Hack Squat	12, 10, 8	12, 10, 8	10, 8, 6, 12	10, 8, 6, 12
Step Up w/ DBs	12, 10, 8	12, 10, 8	10, 8, 6, 12	10, 8, 6, 12
DB RDL	12, 10, 8	12, 10, 8	10, 8, 6, 12	10, 8, 6, 12
Weighted Back Extnesion	12, 10, 8	12, 10, 8	10, 8, 6, 12	10, 8, 6, 12

For the high bar close stance squats, We are trying to do for your legs what the close-grip bench is were trying to do to your triceps. We're doing this to disadvantage of the knee and increase some development in the quads. We are hyper fixating on the "push" that is so important in any squatting movement. Your squats should aim to emulate what looks like a standing leg press.

Some of you may have issues getting into a good position if you aren't very mobile or experienced as a squatter or if you have very long legs. That's okay; your mission here is just to have your feet a bit closer than you normally do and push your knees forward just a bit more. Even if it doesn't look like your favorite powerlifter's crispy-clean high bar stance, the point is that it's different from what you are used to.

I find that it helps to do 5 to 10 minutes of stretching to get into position before these. Spend some time with your toe up on the edge of a squat rack, driving your heel forward into it to loosen your calves up. Get your quads, your hamstrings and your glutes loosened up and you'll find you have an easier time getting the range of motion you need to get the most out of this movement.

Yes, deep stretching will slightly reduce your ability the produce maximal amounts of force. Good thing we aren't here to produce maximal amounts of force.

We are here to get good in positions we suck at.

So don't use a hypothetical 3% difference in force output as a reason for slacking on basic body maintenance.

I also recommend elevating your heels. You can use a mat or piece of plywood under your heels, a small weight plate or you can invest in lifting shoes.

BLOCK 3

Day 1	Week 9 (RPE 7)	Week 10 (RPE 8)	Week 11 (RPE 8)	Week 12 (RPE 9)
Push Press	Top 5, 3x8, 1x15	Top 5, 3x8, 1x15	Top 3, 3x6, 1x12	Top 3, 3x6, 1x12
Seated Military Press	5, 8, 12, 15	5, 8, 12, 15	5, 8, 12, 15	5, 8, 12, 15
Weighted Dips	5, 8, 12, 15	5, 8, 12, 15	5, 8, 12, 15	5, 8, 12, 15
Skull Crusher	3x8	3x8	3x8	3x8
V-Bar Pressdown	3x12	3x12	3x12	3x12

Now we're in Block 3, This is the culmination of the entire program and what I think of as being more of a generic long-term powerbuilding split. The idea behind powerbuilding is somewhat in line with concurrent training in that we are training multiple different thresholds qualities all at once, instead of separating them into two distinctly different blocks.

So you are doing heavy overloaded movements to condition your nervous system to take off the governor and unleash Hell. You are doing a whole host of compound movements for high-volume and to high fatigue to create a brutal muscle building stress. And you are implementing all of the same isolation movements done for crazy amounts of work with brutal fatigue techniques that pro-bodybuilders use in order to make sure that your physique is well rounded and no stone is unturned.

Enjoy the overload movements here. They are a lot of fun and, because they are new, you stand to make a lot of progress quickly. The people who are going to do the best here are the ones who get excited to master these new positions and move some damn weight. Push presses are fantastic for overloading the upper body because, not only are you using a bit of leg drive to get to wait moving, but you are overloading the upper body in the context of standing on your own two feet. It's really hard to do that for your upper body without rigging up a bunch of pain in the ass bands and chains.

Don't go crazy with obsessing over technique here; if you are new to this, just practice getting a small bit of a knee dip-and-drive to get the bar going and then work on pushing through as fast as you can. Every rep and every set that you do will go off better and more efficiently until you're handling ten or even twenty percent over your strict press max for reps.

This equals so much work done with so much more weight than you're used to that the growth tends to be frightening.

Day 2	Week 9 (RPE 7)	Week 10 (RPE 8)	Week 11 (RPE 8)	Week 12 (RPE 9)
13" Deadlift	Top 5, 3x8, 1x15	Top 5, 3x8, 1x15	Top 3, 3x6, 1x12	Top 3, 3x6, 1x12
Good Morning	5, 8, 12, 15	5, 8, 12, 15	5, 8, 12, 15	5, 8, 12, 15
Step Ups w/ DBs	3x8	3x8	3x8	3x8
Weighted Back Extension	3x12	3x12	3x12	3x12

Elevated deadlifts are another favorite of mine for getting the nervous system dialed in. Mechanically, you are just stronger from a higher pick. This movement gets a little weird though because other factors can actually make you weaker here. Some of you might notice that by putting the bar up you sacrifice the leg drive that you are used to relying on to get the deadlift moving off the ground. Now, after all of the Romanian deadlifts and stiff-legged deadlifts, you should find that your hip extension power is on another level here. But you still might find this to be an awkward sticky spot.

Even though this is an overload movement, the name of the game with unfamiliar positions is still to do them long enough to get good at them. As you get better from this height you will find that you can handle much more weight for more reps then you could from the floor and that overload represents a new stress that your body will have no choice but to respond to.

Good mornings are another favorite of mine. I actually prefer these with a safety bar the tax the upper back and midsection or a cambered-bar to put the stress more in the hips and hamstrings. Straight bars are perfectly fine, they just ride a bit more uncomfortably, so if you have access to another bar I recommend using that. This is another one where it's easy to overthink technique because you don't have an obvious endpoint. I used to obsess over whether or not I was deep enough or if I was shorting my movement. You can set the pins up at the start if you want to try to practice proper depth but I find that just visualizing what the bottom position of a Romanian deadlift feels like is the easiest way to gauge where proper depth is.

And by now you are weighted back extensions should be requiring An amount of weight that makes holding onto plates and unviable option. When people start eagerly sharing their results from this program I am going to look past your press, squat and deadlift numbers and ask, "what was your heaviest set with weighted back extensions?".

Day 3	Week 9 (RPE 7)	Week 10 (RPE 8)	Week 11 (RPE 8)	Week 12 (RPE 9)
Pendlay Row	Top 5, 3x8, 1x15	Top 5, 3x8, 1x15	Top 3, 3x6, 1x12	Top 3, 3x6, 1x12
Chest Supported T-Bar Row	5, 8, 12, 15	5, 8, 12, 15	5, 8, 12, 15	5, 8, 12, 15
Behind the Neck Pulldown	3x8	3x8	3x8	3x8
Barbell Curl	5, 8, 12, 15	5, 8, 12, 15	5, 8, 12, 15	5, 8, 12, 15
Alternating DB Curl	3x8	3x8	3x8	3x8

We spent a good amount of time doing strict bent rows so now we are switching to pendlay rows to put a little bit of body English on to the movement. This is a more explosive version of a row although you should still be staying pretty bent over and it remove the eccentric which actually allows a lot more volume to be done without impairing recovery.

I'm a big fan of pendlay and power rows in the right context but not as the sole method for developing the upper back. All of the work you did in the first 8 weeks has more than earned you the right to have some fun with this movement. For the remaining back exercises avoid Sway and use tempo. I find the combining powerful overloaded movements with slower smaller controlled movements is just a fantastic way to gain strength and size.

Day 4	Week 9 (RPE 7)	Week 10 (RPE 8)	Week 11 (RPE 8)	Week 12 (RPE 9)
Wide Bench Press	Top 5, 3x8, 1x15	Top 5, 3x8, 1x15	Top 3, 3x6, 1x12	Top 3, 3x6, 1x12
Close Grip Floor Press	5, 8, 12, 15	5, 8, 12, 15	5, 8, 12, 15	5, 8, 12, 15
Neutral Grip DB Press	3x8	3x8	3x8	3x8
Seated Dip Machine	5, 8, 12, 15	5, 8, 12, 15	5, 8, 12, 15	5, 8, 12, 15
Rope Pressdown	3x8	3x8	3x8	3x8

Widee bench may not necessarily feel like an overload movement but, just like with the elevated dead lift, the limited range of motion is where the benefit is here. So don't worry if you're not handling more weight than you typically do with your most comfortable bench setup. As an added bonus to squeeze a little bit more out of this movement, I would recommend doing them with a short pause. That will make it a little bit harder so you can get more out of whatever weight you are using but will also save your pec insertions from the shock they would otherwise experience by doing a bunch of explosive bounced reps with a very wide grip.

If you can get your starting power off the chest higher in this awkward position, then you are going to be due to hit some nasty numbers by the time you grab the bar with your comfortable grip. We're not going super wide here, like hands out to the collars; this is just 3 to 4 inches wider than where you are normally comfortable grabbing the bar.

Floor presses or another movement I really like for increasing load, especially with a close-grip. Just make sure you have a spotter. Trust me when I say but you don't want to get stuck in a floor press with no one around to grab the bar from you.

Day 5	Week 9 (RPE 7)	Week 10 (RPE 8)	Week 11 (RPE 8)	Week 12 (RPE 9)
Low Bar, Wide Stance Squat	Top 5, 3x8, 1x15	Top 5, 3x8, 1x15	Top 3, 3x6, 1x12	Top 3, 3x6, 1x12
Front Squat	5, 8, 12, 15	5, 8, 12, 15	5, 8, 12, 15	5, 8, 12, 15
Single Leg Press	5, 8, 12, 15	5, 8, 12, 15	5, 8, 12, 15	5, 8, 12, 15
Leg Extension	3x8	3x8	3x8	3x8

This workouts going to feel like a walk in the park after the other stuff that you've gone through leading up to this block. Four exercises done for three to five set each is way beyond what most strength aficionados will do on lower body day. But To you this is such a reduction in workload that you can almost call it a vacation. Don't sleep on it though each set should come with a substantial amount of effort.

The wide stance squats are are overload movement and after all of the Quad dominant work we've been doing this is our opportunity to put some stress back on our hips and use them to hoist the heaviest poundages. It will take some tweaking to get comfortable with your wide stance squat so good thing you have a lot of sets to practice. I recommend letting the bar ride a little bit lower on your rear delts, pointing your toes out to the side just a bit and pushing your knees out to the side to make way for your hips to sink in between them.. As Ed Coan says, "Spread your taint".

When you get in your groove here the movement should feel very Compact and quick like the Reps you knock off in a leg press. Hips back hips forward hips back hips forward. I also find it getting good in this position provides a ton of carry over to your deadlift strength off the floor.

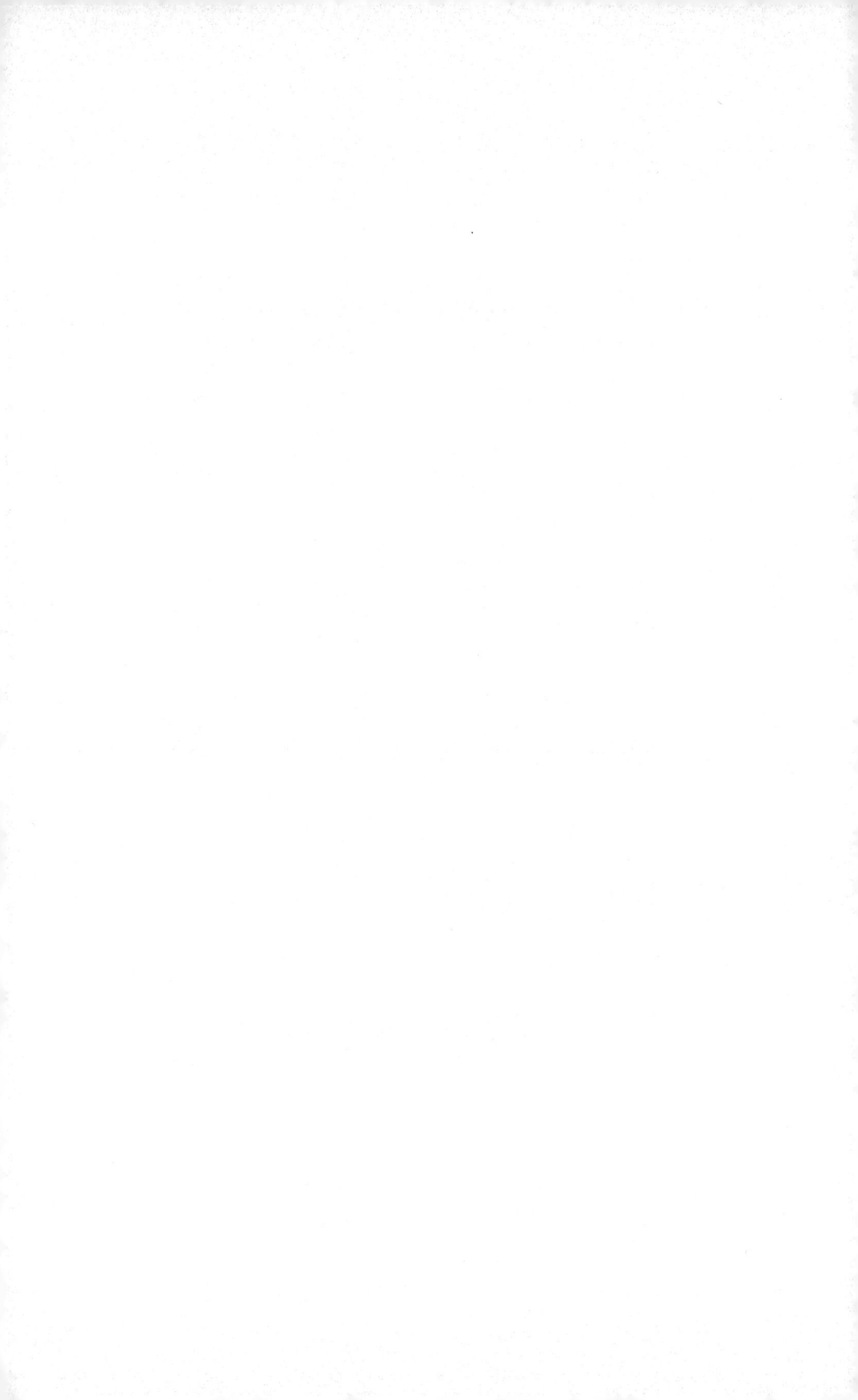

4 DAY SPLIT

To move the 5-day Kong split to 4 days, we moved the back work to lower body day and paired the bicep work with tricep work using supersets. This is actually a very effective way to get this work in and is probably going to work better for most people with a day job and family obligations. The supersets fit very nicely into the goal of this program, which is to expose you to a lot of work and adapt to you to a lot of fatigue.

BLOCK 1

	Week 1		Week 2		Week 3		Week 4	
Day 1								
JM Press to Hammer Curl	3x15	RPE 7	4x12	RPE 5, 7, 10, 10	5x12	RPE 5, 7, 10, 10, 10	5x10	RPE 5, 7, 10, 10, 10
V Handle Pressdown to Cable Curl	3x20	RPE 7	4x15	RPE 5, 7, 10, 10	4x15	RPE 5, 7, 10	4x12	RPE 5, 7, 10, 10
Front Raise w/ DBs	2x15	RPE 7	3x12	RPE 5, 7, 10	4x12	RPE 5, 7, 10, 10, 10	4x10	RPE 5, 7, 10, 10
Upright Row	2x15	RPE 7	3x12	RPE 5, 7, 10	3x12	RPE 5, 7, 10	3x10	RPE 5, 7, 10
Barbell Incline	2x15	RPE 7	3x12	RPE 5, 7, 10	3x12	RPE 5, 7, 10	3x10	RPE 5, 7, 10
Machine Chest Press	2x15	RPE 7	3x12	RPE 5, 7, 10	3x12	RPE 5, 7, 10	3x10	RPE 5, 7, 10
Cable Crossover	2x20	RPE 7	3x15	RPE 5, 7, 10	3x15	RPE 5, 7, 10	3x12	RPE 5, 7, 10
Day 2								
Hamstring Curl	2x20	RPE 7	3x15	RPE 5, 7, 10	3x15	RPE 5, 7, 10	3x12	RPE 5, 7, 10
Leg Press to Romanian Deadlift	2x15	RPE 7	3x12	RPE 5, 7, 10	3x12	RPE 5, 7, 10	3x10	RPE 5, 7, 10
Walking Lunge w/ DBs to Leg Extension	2x12/12	RPE 7	3x12/1	RPE 5, 7, 10	3x12/12	RPE 5, 7, 10	3x10/10	RPE 5, 7, 10
One Arm DB Row	2x20	RPE 7	3x15	RPE 5, 7, 10	3x15	RPE 5, 7, 10	3x12	RPE 5, 7, 10
Lat Pulldown	2x15	RPE 7	3x12	RPE 5, 7, 10	4x12	RPE 5, 7, 10, 10	4x10	RPE 5, 7, 10, 10
Day 3								
Barbell Curl to Dips	3x15	RPE 7	4x12	RPE 5, 7, 10, 10	5x12	RPE 5, 7, 10, 10, 10	5x10	RPE 5, 7, 10, 10, 10
Alternating DB Curl to Rope Pressdown	3x15	RPE 7	4x12	RPE 5, 7, 10, 10	5x12	RPE 5, 7, 10, 10, 10	5x10	RPE 5, 7, 10, 10, 10
Wide Grip Bench Press	2x15	RPE 7	3x12	RPE 5, 7, 10	3x12	RPE 5, 7, 10	3x10	RPE 5, 7, 10
DB Incline Press	2x15	RPE 7	3x12	RPE 5, 7, 10	3x12	RPE 5, 7, 10	3x10	RPE 5, 7, 10
Behind the Neck Press	2x15	RPE 7	3x12	RPE 5, 7, 10	4x12	RPE 5, 7, 10, 10	4x10	RPE 5, 7, 10, 10
One Arm Lateral Raise w/ Cables	2x15	RPE 7	3x12	RPE 5, 7, 10	3x12	RPE 5, 7, 10	3x10	RPE 5, 7, 10
Day 4								
Squat	2x15	RPE 7	3x12	RPE 5, 7, 10	4x12	RPE 5, 7, 10, 10	4x10	RPE 5, 7, 10, 10
Weighted Back Extension to Leg Extension	2x15	RPE 7	3x12	RPE 5, 7, 10	3x12	RPE 5, 7, 10	3x10	RPE 5, 7, 10
Single Leg Press to Hamstring Curl	2x15	RPE 7	3x12	RPE 5, 7, 10	3x12	RPE 5, 7, 10	3x10	RPE 5, 7, 10
Hamstring Curl	2x15	RPE 7	3x12	RPE 5, 7, 10	4x12	RPE 5, 7, 10, 10	4x10	RPE 5, 7, 10, 10
Cable Row	2x15	RPE 7	3x12	RPE 5, 7, 10	3x12	RPE 5, 7, 10	3x10	RPE 5, 7, 10
High Machine Row	2x15	RPE 7	3x12	RPE 5, 7, 10	3x12	RPE 5, 7, 10	3x10	RPE 5, 7, 10

BLOCK 2

	Week 1	RPE 7	Week 2	RPE 8	Week 3	RPE 8	Week 4	RPE 9
Day 1								
Seated Military Press	12, 10, 8, 5, 12		10, 8, 5, 3, 12		10, 6, 5, 3, 8, 12		8, 5, 3, 5, 8, 12	
DB Shoulder Press	12 , 10 , 8		12 , 10 , 8		10, 8, 6, 12		10, 8, 6, 12	
DB Lateral Raise	12 , 10 , 8		12 , 10 , 8		10, 8, 6, 12		10, 8, 6, 12	
Dips to Preacher Curl	12 , 10 , 8		12 , 10 , 8		10, 8, 6, 12		10, 8, 6, 12	
Skull Crusher to Barbell Curl	12 , 10 , 8		12 , 10 , 8		10, 8, 6, 12		10, 8, 6, 12	
V-Bar Pressdown to Cable Curl	12 , 10 , 8		12 , 10 , 8		10, 8, 6, 12		10, 8, 6, 12	
Day 2								
Stiff Leg Deadlift	12, 10, 8, 5, 12		10, 8, 5, 3, 12		10, 8, 5, 3, 8, 12		8, 5, 3, 5, 8, 12	
Bent Barbell Row	12, 10, 8, 5, 12		10, 8, 5, 3, 12		10, 8, 5, 3, 8, 12		8, 5, 3, 5, 8, 12	
Weighted Back Extension to Bulgarian Split Squat	12 , 10 , 8		12 , 10 , 8		10, 8, 6, 12		10, 8, 6, 12	
Leg Press	12 , 10 , 8		12 , 10 , 8		10, 8, 6, 12		10, 8, 6, 12	
Hamstring Curl to Leg Extension	12 , 10 , 8		12 , 10 , 8		10, 8, 6, 12		10, 8, 6, 12	
One Arm Lat Pulldown	12 , 10 , 8		12 , 10 , 8		10, 8, 6, 12		10, 8, 6, 12	
Day 3								
Close Grip Bench Press	12, 10, 8, 5, 12		10, 8, 5, 3, 12		10, 8, 5, 3, 8, 12		8, 5, 3, 5, 8, 12	
Wide Grip Incline Bench	12 , 10 , 8		12 , 10 , 8		10, 8, 6, 12		10, 8, 6, 12	
Machine Chest Press	12 , 10 , 8		12 , 10 , 8		10, 8, 6, 12		10, 8, 6, 12	
DB Fly	12 , 10 , 8		12 , 10 , 8		10, 8, 6, 12		10, 8, 6, 12	
Seated Dip Machine to Barbell Curl	12 , 10 , 8		12 , 10 , 8		10, 8, 6, 12		10, 8, 6, 12	
2 Hand DB Overhead Tricep Extension to Hammer Curl	12 , 10 , 8		12 , 10 , 8		10, 8, 6, 12		10, 8, 6, 12	
Day 4								
Hi Bar Close-Stance Squat	12, 10, 8, 5, 12		10, 8, 5, 3, 12		10, 8, 5, 3, 8, 12		8, 5, 3, 5, 8, 12	
Machine Hack Squat	12 , 10 , 8		12 , 10 , 8		10, 8, 6, 12		10, 8, 6, 12	
Step Up w/ DBs to DB RDL	12 , 10 , 8		12 , 10 , 8		10, 8, 6, 12		10, 8, 6, 12	
Weighted Back Extension to DB Pullover	12 , 10 , 8		12 , 10 , 8		10, 8, 6, 12		10, 8, 6, 12	
Close Grip Lat Pulldown	12 , 10 , 8		12 , 10 , 8		10, 8, 6, 12		10, 8, 6, 12	
Wide Grip Cable Row	12 , 10 , 8		12 , 10 , 8		10, 8, 6, 12		10, 8, 6, 12	

BLOCK 3

	Week 1	RPE 7	Week 2	RPE 8	Week 3	RPE	Week 4	RPE 9
Day 1								
Push Press	Top 5, 3x8, 1x15		Top 5, 3x8, 1x12		Top 3, 3x6, 1x12		Top 1, 3x6, 1x10	
Seated Military Press	5, 8, 12, 15		5, 8, 12, 15		5, 8, 12, 15		5, 8, 12, 15	
Weighted Dips to Barbell Curl	5, 8, 12, 15		5, 8, 12, 15		5, 8, 12, 15		5, 8, 12, 15	
Skull Crusher to Incline DB Curl	3x8		3x8		3x8		3x8	
V-Bar Pressdown to Close Grip Cable Curl	3x12		3x12		3x12		3x12	
Day 2								
13" Deadlift	Top 5, 3x8, 1x15		Top 5, 3x8, 1x12		Top 3, 3x6, 1x12		Top 1, 3x6, 1x10	
Pendlay Row	Top 5, 3x8, 1x15		Top 5, 3x8, 1x12		Top 3, 3x6, 1x12		Top 1, 3x6, 1x10	
Good Morning w/ Pause (2 count)	5, 8, 12, 15		5, 8, 12, 15		5, 8, 12, 15		5, 8, 12, 15	
to Chest Supported T-Bar Row	5, 8, 12, 15		5, 8, 12, 15		5, 8, 12, 15		5, 8, 12, 15	
Weighted Back Extension	3x8		3x8		3x8		3x8	
to Behind the Neck Pulldown	3x12		3x12		3x12		3x12	
Step Ups w/ DBs	3x8		3x8		3x8		3x8	
Day 3								
Wide Bench Press	Top 5, 3x8, 1x15		Top 5, 3x8, 1x12		Top 3, 3x6, 1x12		Top 1, 3x6, 1x10	
Close Grip Floor Press	5, 8, 12, 15		5, 8, 12, 15		5, 8, 12, 15		5, 8, 12, 15	
Neutral Grip DB Press	3x8		3x8		3x8		3x8	
Seated Dip Machine to Alternating DB Curl	5, 8, 12, 15		5, 8, 12, 15		5, 8, 12, 15		5, 8, 12, 15	
Rope Pressdown to Rope Cable Curl	3x12		3x12		3x12		3x12	
Day 4								
Low Bar Wide-Stance Squat	Top 5, 3x8, 1x15		Top 5, 3x8, 1x12		Top 3, 3x6, 1x12		Top 1, 3x6, 1x10	
Front Squat	5, 8, 12, 15		5, 8, 12, 15		5, 8, 12, 15		5, 8, 12, 15	
to Chin Ups	4xF		4xF		4xF		4xF	
Single Leg Extension to Single Leg Press	3x8		3x8		3x8		3x8	
Cable Row	3x12		3x12		3x12		3x12	

HOME GYM 1
No Machines

Before the program was even released, I got a ton of requests for options to run this in a home gym where there isn't a wide selection of machines available. For these modifications, I decided to write them in a 4-day split because we have less movement options to work with. This first example just eliminates the machines, so anybody with a home gym that has a rack, bench a barbell and dumbbells is going to be able to make this work.

I gave substitutions for exercises that I thought best mimicked what the original exercise selection was going for but, as I've said a few times by now, specific exercise selection isn't going to matter here so much. As long as you are trading like-for-like, the spirit of the program is preserved.

BLOCK 1

	Week 1		Week 2		Week 3		Week 4	
Day 1								
JM Press to Hammer Curl	3x15	RPE 7	4x12	RPE 5, 7, 10, 10	5x12	RPE 5, 7, 10, 10, 10	5x10	RPE 5, 7, 10, 10, 10
Inverted Skull Crusher to Concentration Curl	3x20	RPE 7	4x15	RPE 5, 7, 10, 10	4x15	RPE 5, 7, 10	4x12	RPE 5, 7, 10, 10
Front Raise w/ DBs	2x15	RPE 7	3x12	RPE 5, 7, 10	4x12	RPE 5, 7, 10, 10, 10	4x10	RPE 5, 7, 10, 10
Upright Row	2x15	RPE 7	3x12	RPE 5, 7, 10	3x12	RPE 5, 7, 10	3x10	RPE 5, 7, 10
Barbell Incline	2x15	RPE 7	3x12	RPE 5, 7, 10	3x12	RPE 5, 7, 10	3x10	RPE 5, 7, 10
Guillotine Bench Press	2x15	RPE 7	3x12	RPE 5, 7, 10	3x12	RPE 5, 7, 10	3x10	RPE 5, 7, 10
DB Chest Fly (attach mini band if available)	2x20	RPE 7	3x15	RPE 5, 7, 10	3x15	RPE 5, 7, 10	3x12	RPE 5, 7, 10
Day 2								
Glute Bridge (feet elevated on bench)	2x20	RPE 7	3x15	RPE 5, 7, 10	3x15	RPE 5, 7, 10	3x12	RPE 5, 7, 10
Sissy Squat to Romanian Deadlift	2x15	RPE 7	3x12	RPE 5, 7, 10	3x12	RPE 5, 7, 10	3x10	RPE 5, 7, 10
Walking Lunge w/ DBs	2x12/12	RPE 7	3x12/12	RPE 5, 7, 10	3x12/12	RPE 5, 7, 10	3x10/10	RPE 5, 7, 10
to Nordic Leg Extension	2x6		3x6		3x8		3x10	
One Arm DB Row	2x20	RPE 7	3x15	RPE 5, 7, 10	3x15	RPE 5, 7, 10	3x12	RPE 5, 7, 10
DB Pullover	2x15	RPE 7	3x12	RPE 5, 7, 10	4x12	RPE 5, 7, 10, 10	4x10	RPE 5, 7, 10, 10
Day 3								
Barbell Curl to Dips (do on bench if no bars)	3x15	RPE 7	4x12	RPE 5, 7, 10, 10	5x12	RPE 5, 7, 10, 10, 10	5x10	RPE 5, 7, 10, 10, 10
Alternating DB Curl to DB Kickbacks	3x15	RPE 7	4x12	RPE 5, 7, 10, 10	5x12	RPE 5, 7, 10, 10, 10	5x10	RPE 5, 7, 10, 10, 10
Wide Grip Bench Press	2x15	RPE 7	3x12	RPE 5, 7, 10	3x12	RPE 5, 7, 10	3x10	RPE 5, 7, 10
DB Incline Press	2x15	RPE 7	3x12	RPE 5, 7, 10	3x12	RPE 5, 7, 10	3x10	RPE 5, 7, 10
Behind the Neck Press	2x15	RPE 7	3x12	RPE 5, 7, 10	4x12	RPE 5, 7, 10, 10	4x10	RPE 5, 7, 10, 10
One Arm Lateral Raise w/ DB	2x15	RPE 7	3x12	RPE 5, 7, 10	3x12	RPE 5, 7, 10	3x10	RPE 5, 7, 10
Day 4								
Squat	2x15	RPE 7	3x12	RPE 5, 7, 10	4x12	RPE 5, 7, 10, 10	4x10	RPE 5, 7, 10, 10
DB Romanian Deadlift to Nordic Leg Extension	2x15	RPE 7	3x12	RPE 5, 7, 10	3x12	RPE 5, 7, 10	3x10	RPE 5, 7, 10
High Step Up to Glute Bridge (feet elevated)	2x15	RPE 7	3x12	RPE 5, 7, 10	3x12	RPE 5, 7, 10	3x10	RPE 5, 7, 10
Good Morning (knees locked)	2x15	RPE 7	3x12	RPE 5, 7, 10	4x12	RPE 5, 7, 10, 10	4x10	RPE 5, 7, 10, 10
Wide Grip Bent Row (back parallel to ground)	2x15	RPE 7	3x12	RPE 5, 7, 10	3x12	RPE 5, 7, 10	3x10	RPE 5, 7, 10
Meadows Row	2x15	RPE 7	3x12	RPE 5, 7, 10	3x12	RPE 5, 7, 10	3x10	RPE 5, 7, 10

Inverted Skull Crushers are a great way to torch your triceps and don't require any weights. Just like an inverted row you are moving your body weight instead of moving an external weight. Do this by putting a barbell in the rack about chest level and grabbing with a close-grip. Walk your feet back behind you until you are on your tiptoes and then perform what looks like an inverted version of a skull crusher.

I actually like to let my head swoop way past the bar until I get a deep stretch to my elbows and triceps. As I push myself up, I squeez hard at the top for a 1 count and then repeat. You're going to notice that the movement isn't difficult during certain phases of the motion. This is perfectly fine because the Deep stretch paired with the hard squeeze at the top pools a lot of blood in the triceps and creates just a metric fuck ton of fatigue. This is an exceptional exercise to substitute machines or free weights.

Guillotine bench presses are another one that few people are aware of. This takes most of the common-sense advice around safe bench press technique and throws it out the window. Knowing that going into this, expect to start with weights that seem ridiculously light.

You're going to grab the bar with a wide grip several inches wider than you normally bench press with. You are going to let your elbows flare out hard to the side and bring the bar down to your neck instead of your chest. Now if this causes substantial pain in your shoulder or aggravates some pre-existing injury, I strongly recommend that you do not push through it. But most people are going to find that with reasonable we selection they can do this movement, which is essentially a chest fly done with a barbell.

This movement is a great one for lighting up the pecs.

For sissy squats, stand with your toes together and your heels off the ground, grab onto a post of the squat rack with one arm (just for stability) and squat down while leaning back and pushing your knees as far forward as possible. The point here is to put as much stress directly in the knee joint as you can. Again, if this causes pain or aggravates some issue don't move into it. But if you progress at a reasonable rate, this should only make your knee joints stronger. It's also a great way to annihilate the quadriceps. As you progress with your free hand you can hold onto a weight plate crossed in front of your chest.

For Nordic leg extensions, you're going to kneel down with the tops of your feet flat on the ground and you are going to lean back as far as possible, essentially doing an overloaded knee extension to bring your self back up to the kneeling position. It takes quite a while to be able to do these with your bodyweight for reps through a full range of motion but it's still an extremely good exercise with a limited range of motion. Just put a bench behind you and start slow, only increasing depth as you feel comfortable and in control.

BLOCK 2

	Week 1	RPE 7	Week 2	RPE 8	Week 3	RPE 8	Week 4	RPE 9
Day 1								
Seated Military Press	12, 10, 8, 5, 12		10, 8, 5, 3, 12		10, 8, 5, 3, 8, 12		8, 5, 3, 5, 8, 12	
DB Shoulder Press	12, 10, 8		12, 10, 8		10, 8, 6, 12		10, 8, 6, 12	
DB Lateral Raise	12, 10, 8		12, 10, 8		10, 8, 6, 12		10, 8, 6, 12	
Dips (bench if no bars) to Incline DB Curl	12, 10, 8		12, 10, 8		10, 8, 6, 12		10, 8, 6, 12	
Skull Crusher to Barbell Curl	12, 10, 8		12, 10, 8		10, 8, 6, 12		10, 8, 6, 12	
One Arm DB Tricep Extension to Concentration Curl	12, 10, 8		12, 10, 8		10, 8, 6, 12		10, 8, 6, 12	
Day 2								
Stiff Leg Deadlift	12, 10, 8, 5, 12		10, 8, 5, 3, 12		10, 8, 5, 3, 8, 12		8, 5, 3, 5, 8, 12	
Bent Barbell Row	12, 10, 8, 5, 12		10, 8, 5, 3, 12		10, 8, 5, 3, 8, 12		8, 5, 3, 5, 8, 12	
Good Morning to Bulgarian Split Squat	12, 10, 8		12, 10, 8		10, 8, 6, 12		10, 8, 6, 12	
Wide Stance Pause Squat	12, 10, 8		12, 10, 8		10, 8, 6, 12		10, 8, 6, 12	
Single Leg Glute Bridge (feet elevated on bench)	3x8		3x12		3x12		3x15	
to Nordic Leg Curl	3x8		3x12		3x12		3x15	
One Arm DB Row	12, 10, 8		12, 10, 8		10, 8, 6, 12		10, 8, 6, 12	
Day 3								
Close Grip Bench Press	12, 10, 8, 5, 12		10, 8, 5, 3, 12		10, 8, 5, 3, 8, 12		8, 5, 3, 5, 8, 12	
Wide Grip Incline Bench	12, 10, 8		12, 10, 8		10, 8, 6, 12		10, 8, 6, 12	
DB Fly to Guillotine Press	12, 10, 8		12, 10, 8		10, 8, 6, 12		10, 8, 6, 12	
Bench Dips to Barbell Curl	12, 10, 8		12, 10, 8		10, 8, 6, 12		10, 8, 6, 12	
2 Hand DB Overhead Tricep Extension to Hammer Curl	12, 10, 8		12, 10, 8		10, 8, 6, 12		10, 8, 6, 12	
Day 4								
Hi Bar Close-Stance Squat	12, 10, 8, 5, 12		10, 8, 5, 3, 12		10, 8, 5, 3, 8, 12		8, 5, 3, 5, 8, 12	
Sissy Squat	12, 10, 8		12, 10, 8		10, 8, 6, 12		10, 8, 6, 12	
Step Up w/ DBs to DB RDL	12, 10, 8		12, 10, 8		10, 8, 6, 12		10, 8, 6, 12	
Cossack Squat to DB Pullover	12, 10, 8		12, 10, 8		10, 8, 6, 12		10, 8, 6, 12	
Underhand Bent Row	12, 10, 8		12, 10, 8		10, 8, 6, 12		10, 8, 6, 12	
Meadows Row	12, 10, 8		12, 10, 8		10, 8, 6, 12		10, 8, 6, 12	

I put Cossack squats in here because there are limited hamstring exercises when you only have access to free weights. Taking a very wide stance and pivoting your body as you squat down stretches the hamstring, especially around the groin, quite a bit. It's going to test your mobility and it's likely going to make you sore. Scale these to your ability.

Many of you are going to need to start out with just your body weight and holding onto a rack for balance. Your goal should be to be able to do these holding a plate in front of you and then eventually with a light barbell across your shoulders. If you can get through a sufficient range of motion in a Cossack squat with a substantial amount of weight, then you can only assume that your mobility and hamstring and groin strain has become exceptional.

BLOCK 3

	Week 1	RPE 7	Week 2	RPE 8	Week 3	RPE	Week 4	RPE 9
Day 1								
Push Press	Top 5, 3x8, 1x15		Top 5, 3x8, 1x12		Top 3, 3x6, 1x12		Top 1, 3x6, 1x10	
Seated Military Press	5, 8, 12, 15		5, 8, 12, 15		5, 8, 12, 15		5, 8, 12, 15	
JM Press to Barbell Curl	5, 8, 12, 15		5, 8, 12, 15		5, 8, 12, 15		5, 8, 12, 15	
Skull Crusher to Incline DB Curl	3x8		3x8		3x8		3x8	
One Arm DB Tricep Ext. to Reverse Curl	3x12		3x12		3x12		3x12	
Day 2								
13" Deadlift	Top 5, 3x8, 1x15		Top 5, 3x8, 1x12		Top 3, 3x6, 1x12		Top 1, 3x6, 1x10	
Pendlay Row	Top 5, 3x8, 1x15		Top 5, 3x8, 1x12		Top 3, 3x6, 1x12		Top 1, 3x6, 1x10	
Good Morning w/ Pause (2 count)	5, 8, 12, 15		5, 8, 12, 15		5, 8, 12, 15		5, 8, 12, 15	
to One Arm DB Row	5, 8, 12, 15		5, 8, 12, 15		5, 8, 12, 15		5, 8, 12, 15	
Side Lunge	3x8		3x8		3x8		3x8	
to Chin Ups	3xF		3xF		3xF		3xF	
Step Ups w/ DBs	3x8		3x8		3x8		3x8	
Day 3								
Wide Bench Press	Top 5, 3x8, 1x15		Top 5, 3x8, 1x12		Top 3, 3x6, 1x12		Top 1, 3x6, 1x10	
Close Grip Floor Press	5, 8, 12, 15		5, 8, 12, 15		5, 8, 12, 15		5, 8, 12, 15	
Neutral Grip DB Press	3x8		3x8		3x8		3x8	
Bench Dips to Alternating DB Curl	5, 8, 12, 15		5, 8, 12, 15		5, 8, 12, 15		5, 8, 12, 15	
DB Kickbacks to Close Grip Barbell Curl	3x12		3x12		3x12		3x12	
Day 4								
Low Bar Wide-Stance Squat	Top 5, 3x8, 1x15		Top 5, 3x8, 1x12		Top 3, 3x6, 1x12		Top 1, 3x6, 1x10	
Front Squat	5, 8, 12, 15		5, 8, 12, 15		5, 8, 12, 15		5, 8, 12, 15	
to Chin Ups	4xF		4xF		4xF		4xF	
Sissy Squat to Step-Up	3x8		3x8		3x8		3x8	
Wide Grip Bent Row	3x12		3x12		3x12		3x12	

HOME GYM 2
Just a Damn Barbell

For you Savages who are committed to building exceptional amount of muscle mass and physical strength using nothing but a barbell then I have something for you. This split is going to look pretty similar to the previous one but the dumbbell exercises have been swapped out for barbell or body weight variations.

BLOCK 1

	Week 1		Week 2		Week 3		Week 4	
Day 1								
JM Press to Barbell Curl	3x15	RPE 7	4x12	RPE 5, 7, 10, 10	5x12	RPE 5, 7, 10, 10, 10	5x10	RPE 5, 7, 10, 10, 10
Inverted Skull Crusher to Reverse Curl	3x20	RPE 7	4x15	RPE 5, 7, 10, 10	4x15	RPE 5, 7, 10	4x12	RPE 5, 7, 10, 10
Front Raise w/ Barbell	2x15	RPE 7	3x12	RPE 5, 7, 10	4x12	RPE 5, 7, 10, 10, 10	4x10	RPE 5, 7, 10, 10
Upright Row	2x15	RPE 7	3x12	RPE 5, 7, 10	3x12	RPE 5, 7, 10	3x10	RPE 5, 7, 10
Barbell Incline	2x15	RPE 7	3x12	RPE 5, 7, 10	3x12	RPE 5, 7, 10	3x10	RPE 5, 7, 10
Guillotine Bench Press	2x15	RPE 7	3x12	RPE 5, 7, 10	3x12	RPE 5, 7, 10	3x10	RPE 5, 7, 10
Wide Grip Pushup	2x20	RPE 7	3x15	RPE 5, 7, 10	3x15	RPE 5, 7, 10	3x12	RPE 5, 7, 10
Day 2								
Glute Bridge (feet elevated on bench)	2x20	RPE 7	3x15	RPE 5, 7, 10	3x15	RPE 5, 7, 10	3x12	RPE 5, 7, 10
Sissy Squat to Romanian Deadlift	2x15	RPE 7	3x12	RPE 5, 7, 10	3x12	RPE 5, 7, 10	3x10	RPE 5, 7, 10
Walking Lunge w/ Barbell	2x12/12	RPE 7	3x12/12	RPE 5, 7, 10	3x12/12	RPE 5, 7, 10	3x10/10	RPE 5, 7, 10
to Nordic Leg Extension	2x6		3x6		3x8		3x10	
Meadows Row	2x20	RPE 7	3x15	RPE 5, 7, 10	3x15	RPE 5, 7, 10	3x12	RPE 5, 7, 10
Barbell Pullover	2x15	RPE 7	3x12	RPE 5, 7, 10	4x12	RPE 5, 7, 10, 10	4x10	RPE 5, 7, 10, 10
Day 3								
Barbell Curl to Dips (do on bench if no bars)	3x15	RPE 7	4x12	RPE 5, 7, 10, 10	5x12	RPE 5, 7, 10, 10, 10	5x10	RPE 5, 7, 10, 10, 10
Barbell Curl to French Press	3x15	RPE 7	4x12	RPE 5, 7, 10, 10	5x12	RPE 5, 7, 10, 10, 10	5x10	RPE 5, 7, 10, 10, 10
Wide Grip Bench Press	2x15	RPE 7	3x12	RPE 5, 7, 10	3x12	RPE 5, 7, 10	3x10	RPE 5, 7, 10
Incline Close Grip Bench	2x15	RPE 7	3x12	RPE 5, 7, 10	3x12	RPE 5, 7, 10	3x10	RPE 5, 7, 10
Behind the Neck Press	2x15	RPE 7	3x12	RPE 5, 7, 10	4x12	RPE 5, 7, 10, 10	4x10	RPE 5, 7, 10, 10
Upright Row	2x15	RPE 7	3x12	RPE 5, 7, 10	3x12	RPE 5, 7, 10	3x10	RPE 5, 7, 10
Day 4								
Squat	2x15	RPE 7	3x12	RPE 5, 7, 10	4x12	RPE 5, 7, 10, 10	4x10	RPE 5, 7, 10, 10
Romanian Deadlift to Nordic Leg Extension	2x15	RPE 7	3x12	RPE 5, 7, 10	3x12	RPE 5, 7, 10	3x10	RPE 5, 7, 10
High Step Up to Glute Bridge (feet elevated)	2x15	RPE 7	3x12	RPE 5, 7, 10	3x12	RPE 5, 7, 10	3x10	RPE 5, 7, 10
Good Morning (knees locked)	2x15	RPE 7	3x12	RPE 5, 7, 10	4x12	RPE 5, 7, 10, 10	4x10	RPE 5, 7, 10, 10
Wide Grip Bent Row (back parallel to ground)	2x15	RPE 7	3x12	RPE 5, 7, 10	3x12	RPE 5, 7, 10	3x10	RPE 5, 7, 10
Meadows Row	2x15	RPE 7	3x12	RPE 5, 7, 10	3x12	RPE 5, 7, 10	3x10	RPE 5, 7, 10

BLOCK 2

	Week 1	RPE 7	Week 2	RPE 8	Week 3	RPE 8	Week 4	RPE 9
Day 1								
Seated Military Press	12, 10, 8, 5, 12		10, 8, 5, 3, 12		10, 8, 5, 3, 8, 12		8, 5, 3, 5, 8, 12	
Behind the Neck Press	12, 10, 8		12, 10, 8		10, 8, 6, 12		10, 8, 6, 12	
Barbell Front Raise	12, 10, 8		12, 10, 8		10, 8, 6, 12		10, 8, 6, 12	
Dips (bench if no bars) to Close Grip Barbell Curl	12, 10, 8		12, 10, 8		10, 8, 6, 12		10, 8, 6, 12	
Skull Crusher to Barbell Curl	12, 10, 8		12, 10, 8		10, 8, 6, 12		10, 8, 6, 12	
French Press to Inverse Curl	12, 10, 8		12, 10, 8		10, 8, 6, 12		10, 8, 6, 12	
Day 2								
Stiff Leg Deadlift	12, 10, 8, 5, 12		10, 8, 5, 3, 12		10, 8, 5, 3, 8, 12		8, 5, 3, 5, 8, 12	
Bent Barbell Row	12, 10, 8, 5, 12		10, 8, 5, 3, 12		10, 8, 5, 3, 8, 12		8, 5, 3, 5, 8, 12	
Good Morning to Bulgarian Split Squat	12, 10, 8		12, 10, 8		10, 8, 6, 12		10, 8, 6, 12	
Wide Stance Pause Squat	12, 10, 8		12, 10, 8		10, 8, 6, 12		10, 8, 6, 12	
Single Leg Glute Bridge (feet elevated on bench)	3x8		3x12		3x12		3x15	
to Nordic Leg Curl	3x8		3x12		3x12		3x15	
Underhand Bent Row	12, 10, 8		12, 10, 8		10, 8, 6, 12		10, 8, 6, 12	
Day 3								
Close Grip Bench Press	12, 10, 8, 5, 12		10, 8, 5, 3, 12		10, 8, 5, 3, 8, 12		8, 5, 3, 5, 8, 12	
Wide Grip Incline Bench	12, 10, 8		12, 10, 8		10, 8, 6, 12		10, 8, 6, 12	
Guillotine Press	12, 10, 8		12, 10, 8		10, 8, 6, 12		10, 8, 6, 12	
to Pushups	3xF		3xF		3xF		3xF	
Bench Dips to Barbell Curl	12, 10, 8		12, 10, 8		10, 8, 6, 12		10, 8, 6, 12	
French Press to Reverse Curl	12, 10, 8		12, 10, 8		10, 8, 6, 12		10, 8, 6, 12	
Day 4								
Hi Bar Close-Stance Squat	12, 10, 8, 5, 12		10, 8, 5, 3, 12		10, 8, 5, 3, 8, 12		8, 5, 3, 5, 8, 12	
Sissy Squat	12, 10, 8		12, 10, 8		10, 8, 6, 12		10, 8, 6, 12	
Step Up w/ DBs to Romanian Deadlift	12, 10, 8		12, 10, 8		10, 8, 6, 12		10, 8, 6, 12	
Cossack Squat to Barbell Pullover	12, 10, 8		12, 10, 8		10, 8, 6, 12		10, 8, 6, 12	
Underhand Bent Row	12, 10, 8		12, 10, 8		10, 8, 6, 12		10, 8, 6, 12	
Meadows Row	12, 10, 8		12, 10, 8		10, 8, 6, 12		10, 8, 6, 12	

BLOCK 3

	Week 1 RPE 7	Week 2 RPE 8	Week 3 RPE	Week 4 RPE 9
Day 1				
Push Press	Top 5, 3x8, 1x15	Top 5, 3x8, 1x12	Top 3, 3x6, 1x12	Top 1, 3x6, 1x10
Seated Military Press	5, 8, 12, 15	5, 8, 12, 15	5, 8, 12, 15	5, 8, 12, 15
JM Press to Barbell Curl	5, 8, 12, 15	5, 8, 12, 15	5, 8, 12, 15	5, 8, 12, 15
Skull Crusher to Barbell Curl	3x8	3x8	3x8	3x8
Inverted Skull Crusher to Close Grip Curl	3x12	3x12	3x12	3x12
Day 2				
13" Deadlift	Top 5, 3x8, 1x15	Top 5, 3x8, 1x12	Top 3, 3x6, 1x12	Top 1, 3x6, 1x10
Pendlay Row	Top 5, 3x8, 1x15	Top 5, 3x8, 1x12	Top 3, 3x6, 1x12	Top 1, 3x6, 1x10
Good Morning w/ Pause (2 count)	5, 8, 12, 15	5, 8, 12, 15	5, 8, 12, 15	5, 8, 12, 15
to Step Up	4x12	4x12	4x12	4x12
Side Lunge	3x8	3x8	3x8	3x8
to Chin Ups	3xF	3xF	3xF	3xF
T-Bar Row	3x8	3x8	3x8	3x8
Day 3				
Wide Bench Press	Top 5, 3x8, 1x15	Top 5, 3x8, 1x12	Top 3, 3x6, 1x12	Top 1, 3x6, 1x10
Close Grip Floor Press	5, 9, 12, 15	5, 8, 12, 15	5, 8, 12, 15	5, 8, 12, 15
JM Press	3x8	3x8	3x8	3x8
Bench Dips to Wide Barbell Curl	5, 8, 12, 15	5, 8, 12, 15	5, 8, 12, 15	5, 8, 12, 15
Skull Crusher to Close Grip Barbell Curl	3x12	3x12	3x12	3x12
Day 4				
Low Bar Wide-Stance Squat	Top 5, 3x8, 1x15	Top 5, 3x8, 1x12	Top 3, 3x6, 1x12	Top 1, 3x6, 1x10
Front Squat	5, 8, 12, 15	5, 8, 12, 15	5, 8, 12, 15	5, 8, 12, 15
to Chin Ups	4xF	4xF	4xF	4xF
Sissy Squat to Step-Up	3x8	3x8	3x8	3x8
Wide Grip Bent Row	3x12	3x12	3x12	3x12

Thank you for purchasing "KONG"!

It is support from readers like you that allow me to create content full-time, and it is IMMENSELY appreciated.

I promise to always offer as much value as possible in whatever I publish, sell or promote.

If you enjoyed "KONG: SAVAGE SIZE IN 12 WEEKS", consider checking out my previous full-length books:

BASE STRENGTH: Program Design Blueprint
4.8 Stars on Amazon: 191 Ratings

PEAK STRENGTH: Competitive Performance Roadmap
4.8 Stars on Amazon: 88 Ratings

SUPERIOR DEADLIFT: Technique, Principles, Programming
4.9 Stars on Amazon: 48 Ratings

All are available at www.empirebarbellstore.com or at the Amazon Kindle store here: https://amzn.to/3GcRw2N

These are also available to Patreon members, along with accompanying spreadsheets!
https://www.patreon.com/alexanderbromley

Made in the USA
Las Vegas, NV
01 April 2023